FOCUS ON BRAIN CANCER RESEARCH

HORIZONS IN CANCER RESEARCH

Volume 1: Prostate Cancer
John N. Lucas (Editor)
ISBN 1-59454-100-0
Volume 2: Trends in Ovarian Cancer Research
A. P. Bardos (Editor)
ISBN 1-59454-023-3
Volume 3: Percutaneous Cryotherapy of Renal Cell Carcinoma under an Open MRI System
Junta Harada, Kazuo Miyasaka and Sajio Sumida (Editors)
ISBN 1-59454-169-8
Volume 4: Focus on Colorectal Cancer Research
Julia D. Martinez (Editor)
ISBN 1-59454-101-9
Volume 5: Focus on Leukemia Research
Rafael M. Romero (Editor)
ISBN 1-59454-093-4
Volume 6: Progress in Bladder Cancer Research
A. M. Mallory (Editor)
ISBN 1-59454-129-9
Volume 7: Trends in Prostate Cancer Research
John N. Lucas (Editor)
ISBN 1-59454-265-1
Volume 8: Tumor Budding in Colorectal Cancer Recent Progress in Colorectal Cancer Research
Tadahiko Masaki (Editor)
ISBN 1-59454-189-2
Volume 9: Trends in Breast Cancer Research
Andrew P. Yao (Editor)
ISBN 1-59454-134-5
Volume 10: Trends in Leukemia Research
Rafael M. Romero (Editor)
ISBN 1-59454-311-9
Volume 11: Liver Cancer: New Research
Felix Lee (Editor)
ISBN 1-59454-182-5
Volume 12: Focus on Lung Cancer
Robert L. Carafaro (Editor)
ISBN 1-59454-082-9
Volume 13: Treatment of Ovarian Cancer
A. P. Bardos (Editor)
ISBN 1-59454-022-5
Volume 14: Focus on Kidney Cancer Research
Kelvin R. Nunez (Editor)
ISBN 1-59454-110-8
Volume 15: Focus on Pacreatic Cancer Research
Maxwell A. Loft (Editor)
ISBN 1-59454-270-8
Volume 16: Peritoneal Carinomatosis from Ovarian Cancer
Kostantinos N. Chatzigeorgiou and John N. Bontis (Editors)
ISBN 1-59454-398-4
Volume 17: Trends in Pacreatic Cancer Research
Maxwell A. Loft (Editor)
ISBN 1-59454-524-3
Volume 18: Trends in Kidney Cancer Research
Kelvin R. Nunez (Editor)
ISBN 1-59454-141-8
Volume 19: Ovarian Cancer: New Research
A. P. Bardos (Editor)
ISBN 1-59454-241-4
Volume 20: Gene Therapy in Cancer
Grace W. Redberry (Editor)
ISBN 1-59454-288-0
Volume 21: Lung Cancer New Research
Robert L. Carafaro (Editor)
ISBN 1-59454-
Volume 22: New Developments in Bone Cancer Research
Catherine E. O'Neil (Editor)
ISBN 1-59454-337-2
Volume 23: New Developments in Breast Cancer Research
Andrew P. Yao (Editor)
ISBN 1-59454-809-9
Volume 24: Trends in Bone Cancer Research
E. V. Birch (Editor)
ISBN 1-59454-346-1
Volume 25: Focus on Brain Cancer Research
Andrew V. Yang (Editor)
ISBN 1-59454-973-7

Focus on Brain Cancer Research

Horizons in Cancer Research
Volume 25

Andrew V. Yang
Editor

Nova Science Publishers, Inc.
New York

For permission to use material from this book please contact us:
Telephone 631-231-7269; Fax 631-231-8175
Web Site: http://www.novapublishers.com

Library of Congress Cataloging-in-Publication Data

Focus on brain cancer research / Andrew V. Yang (editor).
p. ; cm.
Includes bibliographical references and index.
ISBN 1-59454-973-7
1. Brain--Cancer.
[DNLM: 1. Brain Neoplasms. 2. Brain Neoplasms--secondary. WL 358 F652 2006] I. Yang, Andrew V.
RC280.B7F63 2006
616.99'481--dc22 2006000626

Published by Nova Science Publishers, Inc. ✦New York

Contents

Preface

There are two types of brain tumors: primary brain tumors that originate in the brain and metastatic (secondary) brain tumors that originate from cancer cells that have migrated from other parts of the body. Primary brain cancer rarely spreads beyond the central nervous system, and death results from uncontrolled tumor growth within the limited space of the skull. Metastatic brain cancer indicates advanced disease and has a poor prognosis. Primary brain tumors can be cancerous or noncancerous. Both types take up space in the brain and may cause serious symptoms (e.g., vision or hearing loss) and complications (e.g., stroke). All cancerous brain tumors are life threatening (malignant) because they have an aggressive and invasive nature. A noncancerous primary brain tumor is life threatening when it compromises vital structures (e.g., an artery). In the United States, the annual incidence of brain cancer generally is 15-20 cases per 100,000 people. Brain cancer is the leading cause of cancer-related death in patients younger than 35. This new book brings together the leading research in this dynamic area of research.

Pituitary adenomas comprise 10-15% of all intracranial tumors. Microadenomas, measuring <1 cm, are confined into the pituitary fossa, whereas tumors more than 1 cm (macroadenomas) may extend into the surrounding tissues. Pituitary adenomas are mainly indolent tumors, but around 30-40% of them can become locally invasive while a minority can develop an aggressive behavior with early recurrences after surgical resection as discussed in chapter one. In addition, a small subset, approximately 0.2-0.5%, can develop central nervous system and/or distant metastases and are designated as pituitary carcinomas. The majority of pituitary adenomas is associated with excessive hormonal production inducing characteristic clinical syndromes; however, approximately 20-30% of these tumors are non-hormonal secreting adenomas that are mainly diagnosed as space occupying sellar masses.

The management of pituitary adenomas involves medical treatment and/or surgical excision either alone or with radiotherapy particularly for that subset of tumors that are highly likely to develop early and/or repeated recurrences. Knowledge of the biological behavior of these tumors can facilitate their management as it can direct maximum treatment to tumors that are more likely to develop such an aggressive behavior. Although the proliferative rate of these tumors does not necessarily imply aggressiveness, the great majority of tumors that develop an aggressive behavior exhibit high proliferative rates.

Therefore, the proliferative potential of these tumors could assist to the prediction of their behavior and response to treatment, particularly as routine histopathologic findings are not reliable for this purpose.

Ki-67 is a nuclear antigen that is present in G_1, S, G_2 and M phases of the cell cycle. The development of a monoclonal antibody raised against MIB-1 epitope of the Ki-67 antigen has led to the estimation of the Ki-67 Labeling Index (LI: percentage of positively stained nuclei), which can be used as a predictor of the biologic behavior of pituitary tumors. Ki-67 LI of >3% has been shown to correlate with more aggressive tumoral behavior and higher recurrence risk. In several series hormone-secreting and invasive pituitary adenomas and macroadenomas have been shown to have higher Ki-67 LI than hormone inactive, noninvasive adenomas and microadenomas whereas pituitary carcinomas exhibited significantly higher Ki-67 LI. However, as there has been considerable overlap of the Ki-67 values used to discriminate these pathological entities, it is probable that other unidentified processes also determinate tumor behavior. Currently, high Ki-67 LI represents the most reliable indicator of the biologic behavior of pituitary tumors and can be used to identify cases that need to be monitored more closely.

Historically, there have been two opposing hypotheses concerning the pathogenesis of pituitary adenomas; the hypothalamic hypothesis and the pituitary hypothesis. With the recent demonstration of the monoclonality of most human pituitary adenomas, the pituitary hypothesis, which suggests that pituitary adenomas result from the monoclonal expansion of a single adenohypophyseal cell with subcellular abnormalities, has become the more widely accepted concept. Meanwhile, the role of hypothalamic hormones in the development of pituitary adenomas has recently attracted the attention of investigators once again. In order to confirm the role of locally generated growth hormone-releasing hormone (GHRH) for the progression of somatotroph adenomas, the authors of chapter two investigated the expression of GHRH in 25 pituitary somatotroph adenomas immunohistochemically using both conventional avidin-biotin-complex (ABC) method and novel catalyzed signal amplified (CSA) system. In addition, they investigated the expression of GHRH mRNA and GHRH receptor mRNA with in situ hybridization (ISH) using CSA system. The weak immunopositivity of GHRH were observed in only 2 adenomas (8.0%) out of 25 somatotroph adenomas using ABC method. In contrast, 15 adenomas (60.0%) out of 25 somatotroph adenomas were immunopositive for GHRH revealed by CSA system. Very few of non-somatotroph adenomas were immunopositive for GHRH using CSA system. The expression of GHRH mRNA was confirmed using CSA-ISH system in 13 adenomas (72.2%) out of 18 somatotroph adenomas. In 11 adenomas (61.1%) out of 18 somatotroph adenomas, the expression of GHRH receptor mRNA was demonstrated using CSA-ISH system. The demonstration of GHRH and its receptor expression is meaningful in clarifying the autocrine or paracrine regulation of GHRH in GH production and progression of pituitary somatotroph adenomas. Corticotropin-releasing hormone (CRH) expression in corticotroph adenomas, and gonadotropin-releasing hormone (GnRH) expression in human pituitary adenomas were discussed. Such evidence that indicates endogenous expression of hypothalamic hormones and their receptors in the pituitary and human pituitary adenoma cells has ample significance in autocrine/paracrine regulation of pituitary hormone production.

The extracellular space (ECS) of the brain is an important microenvironment of nerve cells and a communication channel between neurons and glial cells. Its composition and volume change dynamically during neuronal activity, development, aging, many pathological states such as ischemia, demyelination or trauma and during neoplastic reconstruction of the tissue. It has been suggested that changes in ECS volume and composition also affect the biological behavior of brain tumors. ECS size and geometry can be accurately determined by the tetramethylammonium (TMA^+) real-time iontophoretic method, which uses TMA^+ as an extracellular marker and follows its diffusion in the ECS by the use of ion-selective microelectrodes as discussed in chapter three. In comparison with unaffected brain cortex, experiments have revealed a dramatic increase in the ECS volume of gliomas, correlating with increases in malignancy. However, the diffusion of small molecules in the enlarged ECS of high-grade gliomas is slowed down due to increased macromolecule content. In contrast to low-grade tumors, where the diffusion of molecules is reduced mainly by the presence of a dense network of tumor cell processes, the increase of ECS diffusion barriers in high-grade gliomas is caused by the overproduction of certain components of the extracellular matrix (ECM), mainly of tenascin. These aberrant or "overproduced" ECM glycoproteins not only stabilize the ECS volume, but also serve as a substrate for the adhesion and subsequent migration of tumor cells through the enlarged ECS. Interestingly, these alterations in ECS volume and structure may hinder the diffusion of neuroactive substances and drugs into the neoplastic tissue. The presence of tenascin in the ECS of the neoplasm correlates significantly with increased malignancy and poor clinical outcome of the disease, which makes its immunohistochemical detection useful as a marker for the aggressive biological behavior of tumors.

The employment of virus therapy to treat human neoplasms has a several decade long history. One such virus that has been explored is the Newcastle Disease Virus (NDV), in particular, a therapeutic product named MTH-68/H, derived from an attenuated oncolytic NDV strain. MTH-68/H therapy has been employed in a number of different neoplasms with success. This success has also been demonstrated in glioblastomas and anaplastic astrocytomas. Glioblastoma multiforme (GBM) is the most common primary brain tumor and is by far the most aggressive form of glial tumors. This neoplasm has a poor prognosis, averaging six months to a year. Four cases, presently described, of advanced GBM and anaplastic astrocytoma were treated with the NDV viral product MTH-68/H after the classical modalities of anti-neoplastic therapy had failed. The results of the authors in chapter four include survival rates of nine and half, to six years, post viral treatment for the surviving patients, and eight years for one patient who has since died, after becoming non-compliant. Against all odds, these surviving patients returned to a lifestyle that resembles their pre-morbid daily routines. They have been able to enjoy good clinical health. These patients regularly received the MTH-68/H viral therapy for a number of years without interruption as a form of monotherapy once the classical modalities failed. The MRI and CT results have revealed an objective decrease in size of the tumors, in some cases the near total disappearance of the mass. There has also been a documented decrease in mass effect following administration of MTH-68/H. Although one of the four patients described here, did succumb to complications of his malignancy, the results are nonetheless extremely promising in that there is not only a decrease in tumor burden but also a return of pre-morbid functioning. It should be stressed that the positive results may be due to the long-term employment of the oncolytic viral therapy. Chapter four seeks to shed light on the background of MTH-68/H with a focus on the possible mechanism of action. There is also a short description of the clinical course of the four cases, as well as of the functional improvement that the patients experienced with the use of MTH-68/H viral therapy after all classical modalities had failed and hope was nearly lost.

Gliomas are the most common type of primary malignant brain tumors in Malaysia. Several ideas have emerged about the genetic alterations occurring in human cancers and how they contribute to tumorigenesis. The role of common genetic alterations in determining the range of individual susceptibility within the population are being increasingly recognized as indicated in chapter five. The accumulation of genetic alterations are thought to drive the progression of normal cells through hyperplastic and dysplastic stages to invasive cancer and, finally, metastatic disease. With regards to that, numerous research has been aggressively carried out, focusing on the potential roles of genes which are important in cell cycle progression as well as apoptotic pathways. The results revealed *PTEN* and *p53* genes mutations to be found in mostly high grade gliomas. Loss of heterozygosity (LOH) and telomerase activities were also found in high grade glioma cases, suggesting that those actions might contribute to brain tumorigenesis in Malaysia especially amongst the Malay population. The identification of genes and pathways involved would enhance our understanding of the biology of this process. It would also provide new targets for early diagnosis and facilitate treatment design for example in developing DNA vaccine as an anti-cancer agent and virus therapy which has shown promise as a cancer treatment in Malaysia.

Proliferative potentials of 127 patients with meningioma were examined according to an immunohistochemical staining method using an anti-Ki-67 monoclonal antibody, MIB-1, for paraffin sections, and the correlations among MIB-1 staining index (SI), histopathological finding, and clinical course of the disease were analyzed retrospectively in chapter six. The mean MIB-1 SI of 50 male patients with meningioma was 5.5%, whereas that of 77 female patients was 2.7%. High MIB-1 SI was observed in younger patients. These age- and sex-related differences in MIB-1 SI were statistically significant. All the patients were divided into 3 groups: 73 patients with non-recurrent meningioma; 21 patients with recurrent meningioma in whom the specimens obtained during the initial surgery were used to calculate the MIB-1 SI; 33 patients with recurrent meningioma in whom the specimens obtained during the surgery for recurrent tumors were used to calculate the MIB-1 SI. The mean MIB-1 staining indices in these patients were 1.6%, 3.6%, and 8.8%, respectively, and there were statistically significant differences among these three groups. Statistical analyses revealed that meningiomas with MIB-1 SI of 3% or higher have significantly high tendency for recurrence in clinical courses, especially in the first 10 year-follow-up periods. Moreover, there is statistically significant correlation between MIB-1 SI and recurrence in each Simpson's grade. Time interval to the next recurrence in recurrent meningiomas is associated with proliferative potential as demonstrated by MIB-1 SI, and a formula of correlation has been proposed to predict the date of the next recurrence. The examination on proliferative potentials of meningiomas using MIB-1 SI is very important for biological and histopathological analyses and the prediction of future recurrence. The mean BrdU labelling index (LI) of recurrent meningiomas was reported to be significantly higher than that of the non-recurrent meningiomas. BrdU LI also can predict the time to re-operation. BrdU LI, MIB-1 SI, and tumor doubling time of intracranial meningiomas have mutual relationship. Many other biological or genetic variables can affect the proliferation of tumors, and nevertheless, BrdU LI and MIB-1 SI are closely related to clinical recurrence or regrowth of meningiomas.

Neoplastic transformation evolves over a period of time involving the progression of cellular immunophenotype (IP) from normal to hyperplastic to dysplastic, and finally, to fully malignant. Superimposed on these changes is the interaction of the initiated cell with its microenvironment, whereby the neoplastically transformed cells, through the regulation or dysregulation of cytoskeletal, integrin, protease and adhesion molecules among others, develop a novel manner of relation with their surrounding microenvironment. Studies of the neuroendocrine-immune network reveal that the hormonal and cytokine milieu plays an important role impacting the growth and dedifferentiation capabilities of cancer cells. This is further affected by the tumor cells themselves inasmuch as they determine and regulate the constitution of their hormonal microenvironment, allowing the most aggressive and invasive of neoplastically transformed cell clones to promote their own growth and dissemination.

Chapter seven details the clinical significance of immunohistochemistry that has developed over the last quarter century. The advancement of monoclonal antibody (MoAB) technology has been of great significance in ensuring the place of immunohistochemistry in the increasingly accurate microscopic diagnosis of human neoplasms, becoming a method of choice in neuropathology. Selected groups of target molecules of great significance in general cancer biology and of particular importance in brain tumors are discussed. The discovery of neoplasm associated antigens (NAAs) has not only made the more accurate diagnosis of human cancer feasible, but has also shed light on the extensive IP heterogeneity of even the most closely linked human malignancies. The identification of disseminated neoplastically transformed cells by immunohistochemistry has allowed for a clearer picture of cancer invasion and metastasis, as well as the malignant evolution of the tumor cell-associated IP. The sensitivity and significance of immunohistochemistry lies not only in the detection of various tumor-associated markers, but also in the use of information gleaned from extensive evaluations of a particular tumor in establishing a functional molecular biological, biochemical and humoral profile of the particular tumor. The elucidation of the steps of the progression of cancer from pre-malignant to invasive and metastatic forms is of utmost importance in the differential diagnosis of neoplasms and in the establishment of appropriate therapeutic regimens. These regimens will certainly begin to take on a more individualized form, targeting combinations of molecular markers in the increasingly more specific and efficacious management of brain tumors.

In: Focus on Brain Cancer Research
Editor: Andrew V. Yang, pp. 1-32
ISBN 1-59454-973-7

Chapter I

Pituitary Tumors: Value of Proliferation Markers in their Histological Assessment

Alexandra F. Stathopoulou, Gregory Kaltsas and George Kontogeorgos*

Departments of Endocrinology and Pathology,
G. Gennimatas General Hospital of Athens, Athens, Hellas

Abstract

Pituitary adenomas comprise 10-15% of all intracranial tumors. Microadenomas, measuring <1 cm, are confined into the pituitary fossa, whereas tumors more than 1 cm (macroadenomas) may extend into the surrounding tissues. Pituitary adenomas are mainly indolent tumors, but around 30-40% of them can become locally invasive while a minority can develop an aggressive behavior with early recurrences after surgical resection. In addition, a small subset, approximately 0.2-0.5%, can develop central nervous system and/or distant metastases and are designated as pituitary carcinomas. The majority of pituitary adenomas is associated with excessive hormonal production inducing characteristic clinical syndromes; however, approximately 20-30% of these tumors are non-hormonal secreting adenomas that are mainly diagnosed as space occupying sellar masses.

The management of pituitary adenomas involves medical treatment and/or surgical excision either alone or with radiotherapy particularly for that subset of tumors that are highly likely to develop early and/or repeated recurrences. Knowledge of the biological behavior of these tumors can facilitate their management as it can direct maximum

* Address for all correspondence: George Kontogeorgos, M.D., Ph.D. Department of Pathology, G. Gennimatas Athens General Hospital, KOFKA Bldg., 1st Floor, 154 Messogion Avenue, GR-115 27 Athens, Hellas; Tel: (011-30) 210 778-4302; Fax: (011-30) 201 778-4302 or 201 770-5980; e-mail: gkonto@med.uoa.gr

treatment to tumors that are more likely to develop such an aggressive behavior. Although the proliferative rate of these tumors does not necessarily imply aggressiveness, the great majority of tumors that develop an aggressive behavior exhibit high proliferative rates. Therefore, the proliferative potential of these tumors could assist to the prediction of their behavior and response to treatment, particularly as routine histopathologic findings are not reliable for this purpose.

Ki-67 is a nuclear antigen that is present in G_1, S, G_2 and M phases of the cell cycle. The development of a monoclonal antibody raised against MIB-1 epitope of the Ki-67 antigen has led to the estimation of the Ki-67 Labeling Index (LI: percentage of positively stained nuclei), which can be used as a predictor of the biologic behavior of pituitary tumors. Ki-67 LI of >3% has been shown to correlate with more aggressive tumoral behavior and higher recurrence risk. In several series hormone-secreting and invasive pituitary adenomas and macroadenomas have been shown to have higher Ki-67 LI than hormone inactive, noninvasive adenomas and microadenomas whereas pituitary carcinomas exhibited significantly higher Ki-67 LI. However, as there has been considerable overlap of the Ki-67 values used to discriminate these pathological entities, it is probable that other unidentified processes also determinate tumor behavior. Currently, high Ki-67 LI represents the most reliable indicator of the biologic behavior of pituitary tumors and can be used to identify cases that need to be monitored more closely.

Introduction

Pituitary tumors comprise 10-15% of all intracranial tumors and are the most common tumors of the sella region. However, their frequency in unselected adult autopsy material ranges between 5% and 20% (Kovacs et al. 1984, Kovacs et al. 1986). These tumors originate from adenohypophysial cells that consist of five main types, depending on their cell origin, and a few subtypes, according to electron microscopic and immunohistochemistry of the produced hormones (Sanno et al. 2003). Pituitary tumors are almost always monoclonal, benign tumors, which usually exhibit a slow growing rate (Herman et al. 1990, Shimon and Melmed 1997, Asa and Ezzat 1998, Clayton et al. 2000). When hormonally active, they can give rise to characteristic clinical syndromes according to the excess of the secreting hormones, such as acromegaly (hypersecretion of growth hormone – GH) or Cushing's disease (hypersecretion of adrenocorticotrophin hormone – ACTH). Non-functioning adenomas are not associated with any hormonal excess and when of small size (less than 10 mm in diameter) most probably represent an incidental finding (postmortem or radiological). Pituitary adenomas may be small lesions confined to the pituitary fossa or tumors with expansive growth to surrounding tissues developing symptoms of an intracranial mass such as visual disturbances, palsies of cranial nerves that pass through the cavernous sinuses and hypopituitarism (Asa and Ezzat 1998). The rare pituitary carcinomas consist less than 0.5% of symptomatic pituitary tumors and their diagnosis requires the presence of metastatic disease inside or outside the central nervous system (Pernicone et al. 1997).

In general, the prognosis of a tumor depends on its growth rate and metastatic spread. Proliferative processes are focused on DNA replication, known as "cell cycle", and are divided in certain phases: G_1, S, G_2, M (mitosis), while quiescent cells belong to G_0 phase. In the majority of human tumors proliferative rates are crucial for the prognosis and future outcome of the disease. Pituitary tumors, although mostly indolent, in approximately 30-40% can exhibit an aggressive behavior, infiltrating surrounding tissues and developing early recurrences after initial surgery. It has been reported that 10-35% of pituitary adenomas can reccur within 4-20 years (16% in 8 years and 35% in 20 years) following initial treatment (Ciric et al.1983, Ebersold et al.1986). Although the proliferative rate of these tumors does not necessarily imply aggressive behavior, aggressive pituitary tumors exhibit high proliferative rates. Estimation of the proliferative potential would be important in their management, which is medical treatment and/or surgical resection with or without radiotherapy. The efficacy of these treatment modalities might be improved by delineating the biological growth mechanisms of these tumors.

Many approaches to estimate the proliferative potential of pituitary adenomas have been tried over the last decades such as mitotic activity, DNA cytophotometry, S-phase fraction, immunostaining for cyclins, inhibitory proteins and uncharacterized proliferation markers. The development of specific monoclonal antibodies made possible the demonstration of antigenic structures, especially cell cycle related antigens, and has provided a rapid and simple approach to measure the growth fractions in tumor histological sections. The immunostaining with monoclonal antibodies has the advantages of not handling radioactive substances, with no requirement of fresh, unfixed tissues, while provides visual assessment of tissue areas with rapid and clear evaluation of viable tumor cells. The method is sensitive enough for small sized specimens accompanied with histological evaluation. Cell kinetics have also been used to evaluate tumor progression and future outcome. However, although the majority of these approaches are reliable for other types of human malignancies, this is not the case in pituitary tumors (Atkin et al. 1979, Nagashima et al. 1986, Meyer and Coplin 1988, Nishizaki et al. 1989, Mellin 1990, Gerdes et al. 1992, Hsu et al. 1993, Kontogeorgos et al. 1996, Turner et al. 2000a).

Histochemical Approaches

Mitoses

One of the oldest and routinely used histopathologic methods of evaluating the biological aggressiveness of human tumors is the assessment of mitotic activity. However, due to the low growth rate of the substantial majority of pituitary tumors this approach is not as reliable. Although mitotic figures are higher in pituitary carcinomas and invasive adenomas in relation to non-invasive adenomas, they remain extremely low; in addition, there is no reliable threshold that can distinguish these three groups of tumors (Thapar et al. 1996a). Nuclear pleomorphism has been described in 71% of pituitary tumors (Pegolo et al. 1995), with the majority of tumors (mostly GH and ACTH secreting adenomas) exhibiting mild nuclear atypias. Although a correlation was found between the presence of nuclear atypia and hormonal secretion, in different tumor subtypes, there was no correlation with respect to invasiveness, mitotic figures, age, gender or tumor size (Kovacs et al. 1986, Scheithauer et al.

1986, Pegolo et al. 1995). Therefore, mitotic activity and nuclear pleomorphism are not ideal indicators of the proliferative potential of pituitary tumors.

Cytophotometry -DNA Ploidy and S-phase Fraction

Cytophotometry is used to determine the relative proportion of certain cell and tissue substances, based on the distinct correlation between absorbance or fluorescence photometry and the respective substance contents. Microscope cytophotometry with image analysis (ICM) and flow cytometry (FCM) systems are supplementary methods for quantitative DNA analysis and cell cycle distribution, each with a typical spectrum of application. ICM is applicable on cytologic and histologic slides, with the possible errors of sampling, due to preselection, and measuring of a low number of cells, while FCM is the additional option of examining cells in single cell suspensions, with the result of high numbers of measured cells and high resolution of DNA histograms, and the possible errors in sampling from the preparations of cell suspensions and measuring of the non neoplastic contaminants (Meyer and Coplin 1988, Mellin W. 1990).

The DNA cytophotometry can successfully determine DNA ploidy, the heterogeneity of DNA stemlines and assess the actual growth fraction, which has some prognostic significance for the future outcome of human tumors. However, one has to take into consideration the fact that cytometric results vary depending on the type of tissue processing (Mellin 1990, Kontogeorgos et al. 1996). In malignant tumors DNA aneuploidy is a sign of unfavorable prognosis and is associated with rapid progression, early metastases, histopathologic growth pattern of poorly differentiated malignant tumor and an overall adverse outcome (Atkin et al. 1979, Auer et al. 1980). The drawback with pituitary tumors is that DNA aneuploidy is not rare, so it cannot be interpreted as a sign of malignancy (Hulting et al. 1989, Mellin W. 1990). The reported frequency of aneuploidy with FCM among pituitary tumors ranges between 0%-55% (Frederickson et al. 1978, Annico et al. 1983, Anniko et al. 1984, Ludecke et al. 1985, Hulting et al. 1985, Fitzgibbons et al. 1988). Some of these studies have reported the highest rates of aneuploidy in prolactinomas (36%-70%) (Ludecke et al. 1985) and GH/Prolactin producing adenomas (80%) (Anniko et al. 1984), and lowest rates in non-functioning adenomas (Anniko et al. 1984). Many studies confirmed these findings and showed no correlation of DNA ploidy with tumor size, invasiveness, age, sex, preoperative hormone levels and proliferative activity, (Anniko et al.1984, Ahyai et al. 1988, Hulting et al. 1989, Nishizaki et al. 1989, Stefaneanu et al. 1990). In a study of Fitzgibbons et al. (1988), no correlation between cell type, mitotic activity and DNA content or between DNA aneuploidy and the clinical outcome was found. The frequency of aneuploidy in pituitary tumors varies, depending on the used criteria for euploidy - aneuploidy; even in the same tumor results differ (Hulting et al. 1985, Ludecke et al. 1985, Hulting et al. 1989) Thus, in these tumors, aneuploidy peak by FCM may not be suggestive of increased likelihood of clinical recurrence, especially when it has been demonstrated that aneuploid pattern can occur in many morphologically benign tumors (Anniko et al. 1981, Anniko et al.1984, Hulting et al. 1985). However, Ludecke et al.(1985) advices continuous follow up of the tumors that have exhibited aneuploidy, because in that study, apart from the confirmation of the previous ones, aneuploidy correlated positively with mitotic index and tumor recurrence. Kontogeorgos et al. (1996), using a high resolution ICA system, have found aneuploid histograms mostly in functioning adenomas compared to nonfunctioning tumors. Further studies also confirmed high association of aneuploid histograms with cytogenetic aberrations of chromosome 11 (Kontogeorgos et al. 1999a). Although DNA ploidy appears to have some prognostic significance, it fails to provide meaningful criteria for therapy planning.

Estimation of S-phase fraction was another approach used to determine the proliferative potential of an individual tumor. The S-phase data with cytometry (intermediate DNA content between that of G_0/G_1 and G_2/M as a marker of S-phase cells) correlate well with the proportions of cells in S-phase, implying that high levels reflect high proliferative activity, suggesting a rapid, and potentially malignant growth. The duration of the cell cycle and the cell turnover, which cannot be estimated by DNA histograms, are critical for the actual growth of a tumor. One drawback of using FCM is that S-phase arrested cells and non-malignant cells are included in the S-phase count and DNA abnormalities without quantitative change in DNA content are not detected. (Meyer and Coplin 1988). However, more reliable results might be obtained when ICM with large numbers of selected intact cells and careful definition of limits to high resolution DNA histograms is used (Kontogeorgos et al. 1996).

Autoradiography with Tritiated (H^3)-Thymidine incorporation into the DNA of replicating cells was initially used for cell kinetics studies, after in vitro incubation of the specimens, to estimate the S-phase fraction of the tumors. Aneuploid tumors exhibited higher thymidine labeling index and S-phase fractions than diploid tumors (Meyer and Coplin 1988). Limitations, such as the potential radiation hazard and the time consuming procedure led to the next step of using the thymidine analogue bromodeoxyuridine (BrdU). The development of a monoclonal antibody (Mab) against BrdU (Gratzner 1982) enabled the in vivo (preoperative intravenous infusion) or the in vitro use of BrdU for S-phase fraction measurements, with the same results as thymidine (Sasaki et al. 1986, Nemoto et al. 1988, Meyer et al. 1993). The BrdU Mab, which is neither radioactive nor myelotoxic, also applied to either tissue sections or single cell suspensions (Hoshino et al. 1986a, Nagashima et al. 1986, Chatterjee et al. 1993). New techniques have been developed to improve immunoreactivity with the use BrdU Mab to label proliferating cells (Nagashima et al. 1985, Sasaki et al. 1986, Tamatani et al. 1995), with rapid results and positive correlation of the labeling index and the proliferative potential of the tumors (Nagashima et al. 1985, Chatterjee et al. 1993).

In many studies of pituitary adenomas, no correlation of S-phase fraction and size, duration of symptoms, ploidy, invasion, age, hormone levels, supra-sellar extension, type of adenoma or tumor recurrence was found (Hulting et al. 1985, Nagashima et al. 1986, Cho et al. 1988, Fitzgibbons et al. 1988, Shibuya et al. 1992), with a wide range of S-phase fraction values (Hoshino et al. 1986b, Ahynai et al. 1988, Ikeda and Yoshimoto 1992, Meyer et al. 1993, Kramer et al. 1994), although there have been some studies that reveal a correlation of the S-phase fraction with ploidy, hormone secretion and more aggressive clinical course (Anniko et al. 1983, Kontogeorgos et al. 1996). However, the limited value of the results on treatment decision led to discontinuation of these techniques.

Further studies tried to correlate the S-phase fraction with nuclear organizer regions (NORs) stained with argyrophilic staining techniques (AgNORs). NORs are located in the secondary constrictions of five acrocentric chromosomes (Denton et al. 1977). They contain genes encoding for ribosomal RNA and take part in the formation of the nuclei, with a linear correlation with S-phase in certain neoplasms (Denton et al. 1977, Stefaneanu et al. 1990). However, no correlation was found between the number of AgNORs and BrdU labeling index and age, sex, duration of symptoms, atypical histological features, clinical aggressiveness and tumor size in pituitary adenomas (Maier et al. 1990, Shibuya et al. 1992). These studies demonstrated a significant correlation of only hormonal secretion (higher in non-functioning adenomas and prolactinomas after treatment with bromocriptine, with no significant correlation with subtypes of functioning adenomas) and recurrent tumors.

Cell Cycle Regulating Molecules

Cyclins and cyclin-dependent kinases (CDKS) are essential for cell cycle regulation in eukaryotes. Cyclins, the regulatory subunits, bind to CDKS, the catalytic subunits, to form active cyclin-CDK complexes. These complexes drive cells through particular phases of cell-cycle, called "check points'', by phosphorylating the unique sets of protein substrates that are essential to achieve transition to the next phase. Cyclins are only present during particular phases of the cycle, due to specific control of their expression. Induction of them requires the presence of growth factors and adherence to extracellular matrix. Their over-expression has been shown to be present in many different tumor types (Jordan et al. 2000, Turner et al. 2000a).

Cyclin D is present in G_0/G_1 phase, normally is growth factor dependent and regulates the transition to S-phase. Disregulation and over-expression, in the absence of growth factors, leads to cell proliferation and may contribute to oncogenesis. In normal pituitary it is absent, whereas in pituitary adenomas is infrequent (less than 10%) but in a large number of cells (Jordan et al. 2000). Cyclin D has found to be overexpressed in non-functioning pituitary adenomas (NFPA), macroadenomas and tumors that recurred following initial treatment, but there was no correlation with tumor invasiveness and pituitary carcinomas (Jordan et al. 2000, Turner et al. 2000a).

Cyclin E occurs in the beginning of G_1, is maximum at G_1/S transition and is degraded in the beginning of the S-phase; it is important for initiation of DNA replication. Cyclins D and E in combination with CDKs regulate G_1 phase, during the division of the cell. Over-expression of cyclin E has been associated with poor differentiation and invasiveness in breast cancer (Keyomarsi et al. 1994). Although cyclin E is positive in a minority of normal and adenomatous pituitary tissues, most frequent in corticotroph adenomas and macroadenomas, there is no evidence to suggest that its over-expression may lead to cell transformation (Jordan et al. 2000, Turner et al. 2000a).

Cyclin A accumulates in late G_1, is maximum in S-phase and degraded in M-phase. An over-expression advances the entry of cells into S-phase, reducing the duration of cell cycle. In other types of tumors it is implicated for early relapse, poorer tumor grading and reduced survival; however, there is no evidence that its over-expression may lead to increased cell proliferation in pituitary tumors. It has only been found marginally over-expressed in macroadenomas and adenomas, which regrow following initial treatment (Turner et al. 2000a, Nakabayashi et al. 2001).

Cyclin B is important for the transition from G_2 to M phase. Its over-expression has been reported in some cancers. In pituitary adenomas over-expression was found in macroadenomas and NFPA that regrow (Turner et al. 2000a). There is no evidence that over-expression of cyclins leads to pituitary tumorigenesis. Maybe this is secondary to another signal that switches on the cell-cycle machinery and leads to increased cell proliferation.

Proliferative Cell Nuclear Antigen (PCNA) is another cyclin that has been investigated over the last years for its role to cell proliferation and its possible participation to tumorigenesis. It is a 36 kD nuclear polypeptide identified as the auxiliary protein of deoxyribonucleic acid polymerase δ (involved in DNA replication); its gene expression correlates with cell proliferation. It is synthesized in the late G_1 and S-phases, decreased in G_2 to very low levels in mitosis and it is undetectable in G_0. High levels of nuclear positive PCNA were found in aneuploid tumors, carcinomas and proliferating compartments of non neoplastic tissues with high S-phase fractions and BrdU Labeling Index (LI); a correlation with mitotic activity was also demonstrated in human solid tumors (Robbins et al. 1987). Hsu et al. (1993) used the Mab 19A2 (monoclonal antibody) against PCNA and showed that normal pituitary exhibited occasional PCNA positivity, whereas high PCNA indices were found in large pituitary tumors, and in adenomas with extrasellar extension and incomplete surgical excision.These factors (high PCNA index, macroadenoma, extracellar extention and incomplete surgical excision) together were found as highly significant positive predictors of tumor recurrence, with the high PCNA index being the major contributor than the others. Each of them was not independently significant. No association was found to tumor subtypes, gender, age, hormone hypersecretion, disease free interval, irradiation or bromocriptine treatment. These tumors exhibited more than 50% positivity to PCNA, some with regional variations, while mitotic cells were faintly labeled. Significant higher PCNA levels were found in recurrent compared to non-recurrent adenomas with 90% of the recurrent tumors exhibiting PCNA positive nuclear fractions greater than 5%. A comparison between the recurrent adenomas and the initial tumor on the same individuals revealed that the PCNA index was higher in the recurrent tumor. Subsequent studies exhibited similar results (Gardour-Edwards et al. 1995, Kawamoto et al. 1995, Nose-Alberti et al. 1998); However, there were also studies that did not confirm those findings (Ekrabullah et al. 1996, Schreiber et al. 1999) and therefore further studies are required to clarify whether there is any correlation of PCNA and pituitary adenomas invasiveness. PCNA index is higher than thymidine or S-phase fraction from FCM DNA histograms, because the observer counts only tumor cells, without measuring the non neoplastic contaminants and because both G_1 and G_2 are detectable instead of only S-phase, as with thymidine labeling (Kurki et al. 1986, Galand and Degraef 1989, Garcia et al. 1989). In rat tissues Muskhelishvilli et al. (2003) showed an absence of significant correlation of PCNA and BrdU indexes, whereas Atkin et al. (1997) compared PCNA with BrdU LI of human pituitary adenoma cell cultures and found a significant association, although PCNA LI was present in high levels. Delgrange et al. (1997) while studying a group of prolactinomas found no correlation between PCNA LI and tumor size, invasion and/or age. The value of PCNA labeling index as a proliferative marker has been considerably questioned because of the variation of detectable levels among different cell types or malignant cells in comparison to normal state, its long half-life, its involvement in DNA repair with staining of cells that are not actually dividing and also due to its dependence on the fixatives and antigen retrieval solutions (Hall et al. 1990, Shivji et al. 1992, Muskhelishvilli et al. 2003).

p53, a 53kD phosphoprotein, is the product of p53 tumor suppressor gene that is located in chromosome 17p13.1 and exerts a central role in the control of cell proliferation. The normal wild type p53 is a protective regulatory element that maintains the integrity of the cellular genome through a variety of yet poorly understood mechanisms. If DNA is damaged, p53 accumulates and switches off replication (induces G_1 arrest, inhibits G_1-S transition, represses transcription of various growth promoting genes) to allow extra time for its repair; if the repair fails, p53 can trigger cell suicide through the induction of apoptosis (Lane 1992). When p53 is mutated its function is lost and there is an induction of alterations that stabilize the protein in transformed cells. p53 mutation is the most frequently genetic mutation identified of human cancers and its accumulation is an unfavorable factor of a wide range of human neoplasms (Levine et al. 1991, Cunningham et al.1992, Hollstein et al. 1994). In normal cells p53 is undetectable by immunohistochemistry, when specific monoclonal antibodies are used.

Pituitary adenomas exhibit an expression of p53 with no relationship to the functional status, but with a significant association with invasive status and metastatic dissemination, mostly related to the presence or absence and not to the density of immunostaining (Thapar et al. 1996b). In one study, Buckley et al. (1994) demonstrated a correlation of p53 with only corticotroph adenomas, invasive NFPA and pituitary carcinomas, but no correlation with non-invasive NFPA, somatotroph adenomas or prolactinomas. Approximately 16% of invasive adenomas demonstrate p53 protein immunohistochemistry whereas pituitary carcinomas may or may be not p53 positive; in contrast, post-mortem normal pituitary is always p53 negative. (Saeger et al. 1999, Gaffey et al. 2002, Harada et al. 2000). Nevertheless, p53 expression is thought to be of prognostic significance in pituitary carcinomas (Hollstein et al. 1994, Thapar et al. 1996b). Suliman et al. (2001) found expression of p53 in 61% of pituitary adenomas, without any correlation of p53 status with invasiveness or tumor size. The differences between those reports are due to lack of methodological standards in the techniques and differences in well validated anti-p53 antibodies, tissue fixation and processing with less sensitive immunohistochemical protocols, variability in designating p53 immunopositivity and small sample size. Being a nuclear protein, p53 gene mutations would be expected to result in nuclear accumulation of the mutated protein; cytoplasmic staining is observed with or without mutations of the p53 gene. Wild p53 protein can accumulate in the cytoplasm following binding to other proteins, such as heat shock proteins, and this probably consists a physiological mechanism of inactivation of the protein by removing it for the site of its action, thus allowing cell proliferation without a mutation altering the normal action (Buckley et al. 1994, Kontogeorgos et al.1999b). Positive p53 protein in pituitary adenomas can thus be interpreted as a sign of invasiveness whereas a negative p53 protein does not necessarily exclude a more rapid or malignant tumor growth. Correlation to growth fractions can be regarded as additional biological information that should alert the clinician and prompt careful postoperative clinical surveillance. The apoptotic LI was shown to be lower in p53 positive tumors and had no correlation with cytoplasmic p53 positive or negative pituitary tumors. The nuclear accumulation was associated with lower apoptotic index, whereas in other types of tumors high nuclear p53 is associated with high apoptotic index (Schlamp et al. 1997, Kontogeorgos et al.1999b). It is probable that the accumulation of p53 in pituitary adenomas is used to counteract another antiapoptotic mechanism that is upregulated or some dysfunction of the wild type, leading, despite its enhanced production, to reduction of its apoptotic action.

Many other inhibitory proteins are under investigation as possible proliferation markers. $P21^{WAF-1}$, a is a cyclin dependent kinase inhibitor and a downstream mediator of p53 function, whereas mdm2 protein, which is induced and binds to p53 in an autoregulatory feedback loop suppressing wild type p53 activity, have not been shown to exert any correlation with pituitary adenoma's size or invasion (Suliman et al. 2001). Bcl-2 is an integral mitochondrial membrane protein, from bcl-2 proto-oncogene, being localized to mitochondria and interfering with programmed cell death; it acts independently to promote cellular division, block apoptosis and give cells a survival advantage (Hockenbery et al. 1990). It also inhibits cell growth (Knowlton et al. 1998). It has been demonstrated that normal pituitary lacks any bcl-2 staining, whereas over 50% of pituitary tumors, particularly NFPA, exhibit positive staining without any significant correlation with adenoma size or type, and also a correlation between high immunostaining of cyclin D and lower bcl-2 staining in tumors that regrow (maybe in another pathway where bcl-2 is down-regulated, leading to reduction of cell differentiation and also survival and aggressive behavior are promoted) (Turner et al. 2000a, Turner et al. 2000b, Harada et al. 2000) In a study of Turner et al.(2000b) a positive association of bcl-2 and angiogenesis was found, but the latter did not exhibit any correlation with tumor regrowth. Sambaziotis et al. (2003) exhibited bcl-2 immunostaining in nontumorous adenohypophysial cells and expression of bcl-2 protein in over half of the pituitary tumors studied, much higher in nonfunctioning adenomas, with a significant inverse correlation to apoptotic labeling index. It is probable that overexpression of bcl-2 presents an early event in pituitary tumorigenesis, leading to indolent tumor growth and cell survival, as its expression is known to inhibit cell proliferation.

Cyclin-dependent kinase inhibitor $p27^{kip-1}$ is a key molecule, regulating G_1 phase of cell cycle by inhibiting Cyclin-CDKs complexes of that phase. Postmortem specimen from normal pituitaries and from normal pituitary tissues resected during adenomectomies exhibit more than 80% expression, while a reduction is noted in pituitary tumors of any type (less than 10% of the tumor cells) (Bamberger et al. 1999). Bamberger et al. (1999) showed that down regulation of p27 is important for cellular proliferation in both malignant and benign neoplasms. In other studies lower expression of p27 was found in pituitary carcinomas than adenomas, especially corticotrophs (Korbonits et al. 2002, Gaffey et al. 2002), and in recurrent adenomas compared to non-recurrent adenomas (Nakabayashi et al. 2001). Other factors have also been investigated over the last years.

DNA polymerase α (Shibuya et al. 1992) was found to be increased in recurrent and invasive adenomas; however, there was no threshold indicative of aggressive behavior.

Telomerase activity was shown to be present only in late recurrences in a minority of adenomas that underwent malignant transformation (Harada et al. 2000).

c-myc protein, closely involved to cell proliferation, was found to be increased in pituitary adenomas and significantly higher in invasive adenomas (Ikeda and Yoshimoto 1992). Recently, Muskhelishvilli et al. (2003) attempted to correlate the quantification of histone mRNA with the S-phase fraction in rat tissues. The synthesis of histones that are restricted to the cells being in the S-phase of the cell cycle were found to be increased 50-fold. Although this could be a precise molecular marker of estimating cells being in the S-phase of the cell cycle, overfixation or RNase contamination of specimens can reduce the signal and affect the accuracy of detection of labeled cells (Muskhelishvilli et al. 2003). Inhibitory proteins of the cell cycle such as p16, DNA topoisomerase IIα, Urokinase, Urokinase Receptor, Urokinase Inhibitor, Tissue Plasminogen Activator and many other proteins or antigens have been investigated during the last years with yet poor results in an effort to find a biologically relevant, prognostically informative marker capable of distinguishing aggressive pituitary tumors from those having a more indolent biological behavior.

Ki-67

Ki-67 antigen, was defined originally by the prototype monoclonal antibody Ki-67, generated by immunizing mice with nuclei of the Hodgkin lymphoma cell line L428. It was first described in 1983 and was named from the city origin (Kiel, West Germany) and the number of the original clone in the 96-well plate. The antibody is of the IgG_1 subclass and is reactive to a nuclear structure, mapped in chromosome 10, present in proliferating normal or tumor cells in late $G_1/S/G_2/M$ phases but not in G_0 and early G_1 phase of the cell cycle. No homology of the protein to any known polypeptide and no link to the known key regulators of the cell division cycle has been found (Gerdes et al. 1984, Brown and Gatter 1990, Scholzen and Gerdes 2000). The Ki-67 protein expression seems to reflect directly a certain physiological state of the cell and is an antigen continuously present during the cell cycle of all cell types with rapid disappearance during the transition from any part of the cell cycle to a non-proliferative state. Ki-67 seems to be a distinct marker to determine the growth fraction of a given cell population, as there is no variance between cells in different phases and its biological half life is 90 minutes. Positivity for Ki-67 does not necessarily means that a cell is actively dividing, but it expresses the potential of the cell to proliferate (Scholzen and Gerdes 2000).

Since Gerdes et al.(1984) introduced the use of Ki-67 as a marker for the assessment of growth fraction with a unique prognostic relevance in human tumors, a considerable amount of literature has been generated. The usefulness of Ki-67 has been established for various types of malignant neoplasms, particularly for neoplasms where conventional histological criteria are difficult to predict their biological behavior (Gerdes et al. 1983, Zuber et al. 1988, Girino et al. 1990). An initial drawback was the limited cross-species reactivity. The production of monoclonal antibodies against recombinant parts of the Ki-67 antigen, true Ki-67 equivalents regarding immunohistochemistry and immunobiochemistry, helped to overcome this difficulty. The MIB-1 clone of Ki-67 mouse anti-human antibody is the equivalent protein in various mammals, whereas the MIB-5 clone of mouse anti-rat antibody is used in rodents (Birner et al. 2001, Muskelishvilli et al. 2003). The Ki-S5 clone of mouse anti-human antibody shows similar reaction pattern as monoclonal mouse anti-human Ki-67 antibody and the TEC-3 clone of rat anti-mouse antibody is for murines, with similar staining pattern with human tissues (Scholzen and Gerdes 2000). Lastly, the clone SP6 of mouse Ki-67 antibody was recently introduced (Lab Vision datafile). It should be however noted that all accumulated information regarded tumor proliferative activity was based on Ki-67, clone MIB-1 antibodies. Therefore, applications of antibodies of other clones provide incompatible results.

Initially Ki-67 antibody and an equivalent monoclonal antibody MIB-2 failed to stain following routine paraffin embedding processes, as the specific epitope they recognized did not survive histopathological fixation. Modified microwave oven pretreatment of paraffin sections, revealed the nuclei staining of the proliferative cell compartment of several tissues with these monoclonal antibodies against the Ki-67 antigen, as it was recognized by all in formalin-fixed paraffin embedded sections (Shi et al. 1991, Gerdes et al. 1992, Gattoretti et al.1992, Scholzen and Gerdes 2000). Until then, Ki-67 antibodies were used only in frozen sections while the PCNA antibody, PC10, had the advantage of being used in formalin fixed paraffin sections (Kubbutat et al. 1994). When the microwave oven procedure was used, antibodies of clones MIB-1 and MIB-3 revealed strong nuclear staining that was identical to that seen with Ki-67 antibody in frozen sections. Moreover, routine decalcification or depigmentation techniques did not alter the immunoreactivity for antibodies of MIB-1 and MIB-3 clones in those paraffin sections (Gerdes et al. 1992, Gattoretti et al. 1992). The microwave oven procedure of formalin fixed paraffin sections is highly reproducible, with low cost, easy to perform in every histopathological laboratory all over the world, applicable to stored sections while no particular technical skill is needed. The main advantages of MIB-1 and MIB-3 clones are the combination of the optimally preserved morphology with strong immunoreactivity, the clear immunoreactivity of products that allows distinction between positive and negative cells even in cases of weak staining and the easy applicability of the method (Gattoretti et al. 1992). However, there are several discrepancies with regard to localization and function of Ki-67 antigen. The former is probably due to different fixation and staining protocols and the inaccessibility of the entire antigen, caused by conformational changes that "mask" the antigen determinant or formation of supramolecular complexes that influence the interaction between the antigen and the antibody (Braun et al. 1988). Therefore, estimation of Ki-67 LI (percentage of positively stained nuclei) requires cautious studies from an expert pathologist who has to exclude from counting other Ki-67 labeled cells, which are included in the histological sections (Figure 1). Endothelial cells in tumors showing high antiangiogenetic activity, reactive stoma fibroblasts and mononuclear inflammatory cells represent the most common nontumorous cell elements. It has also been reported that binding of these antibodies to Ki-67 protein depend on the ionic strength (Bruno and Darzynkiewicz 1992) or the binding of Ki-67 to DNA (Lopez et al. 1994); the intensity of staining is possibly linked to its biological behavior (Scholzen and Gerdes 2000). Ki-67 staining increases in S-phase (Bruno and Darzynkiewicz 1992) with the highest levels obtained in metaphase and anaphase while it starts to decrease in telophase (Braun et al. 1988). After mid-G1 the only localization is the nuclei (Braun et al. 1988, Brown and Gatter 1990, Scholzen and Gerdes 2000). The reasons for unsuccessful determination of Ki-67 function are its relevant small size and the presence of two isoforms, the post-transcriptional modifications, the high susceptibility to protease cleavage and the absence of homology to known molecules (Scholzen and Gerdes 2000). Another practical problem is the heterogeneity of tumoral cell, raising the possibility that a small biopsy may not reflect the predominant proliferation rate of a tumor (Brown and Gatter 1990).

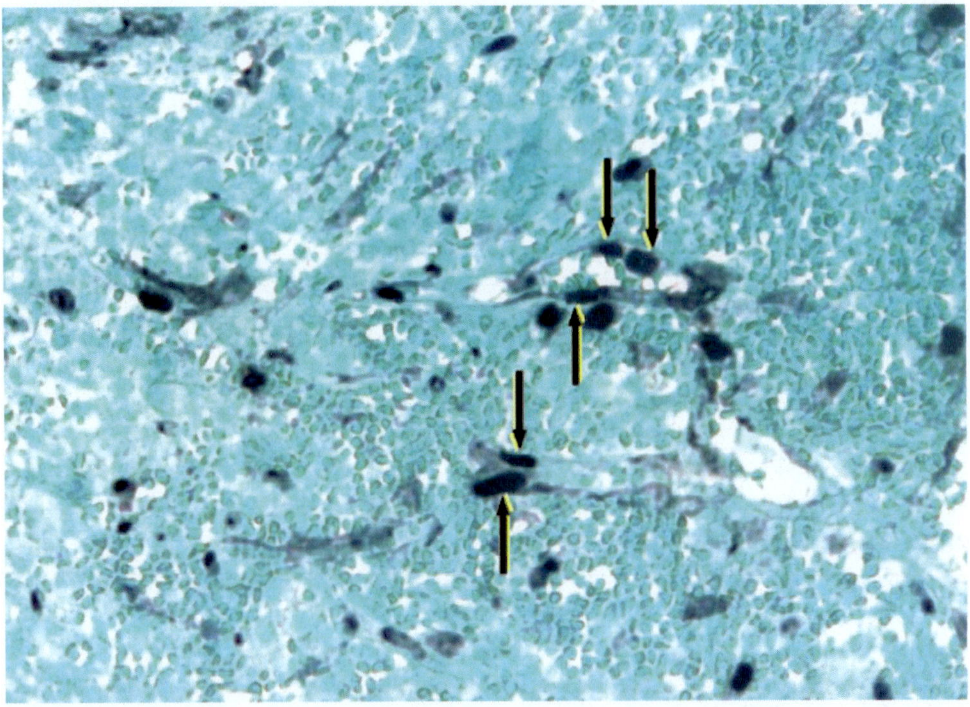

Figure 1. Area of the previous adenoma including sinusoids with Ki-67 positive proliferative endothelial cells, pointed with arrows (ABC 20X).

Pituitary Adenomas and Ki-67

The assessment of a reliable proliferation marker in pituitary tumors that could facilitate their management is very important as although pituitary tumors are considered to be slow growing tumors, a great proportion of them may develop an aggressive behavior and early recurrences. As the estimation of Ki-67 antigen (Figures 2,3) appears to be the best method currently available to determine the proliferative activity of human tumors, many studies over the last years have tried to determine whether an association of this marker with specific characteristics of pituitary tumors, such as tumor size, secretion status, invasion and/or recurrence, exists; this effort has produced several discrepant results. This is possibly due to different techniques and the heterogeneity of pituitary tumors leading to different conclusions regarding the LI, the underestimation of the variability of LI and the fact that the influence of the preoperative treatment has not been considered in many cases.

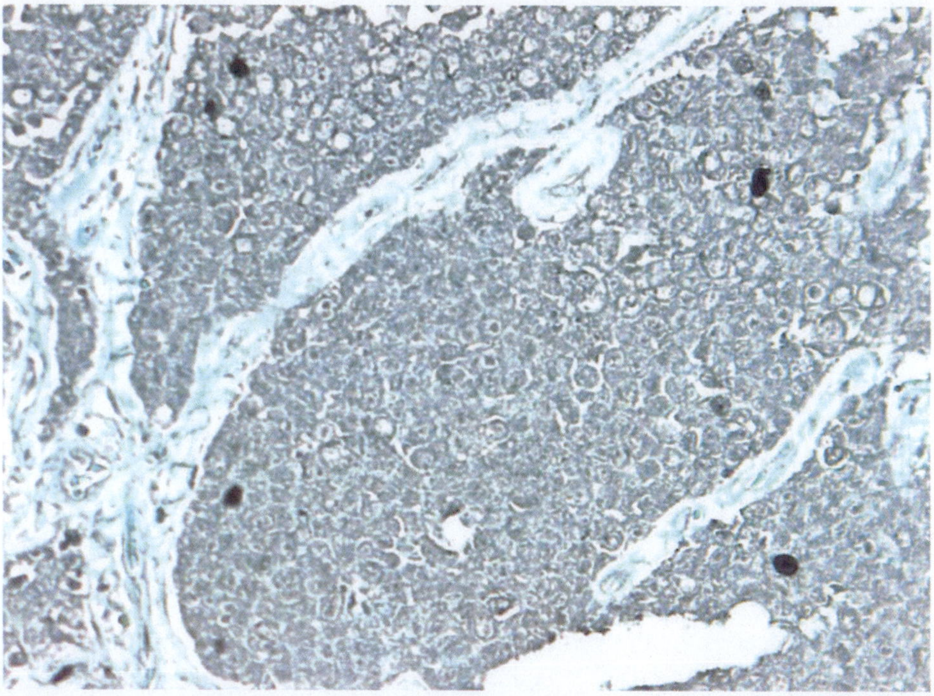

Figure 2. Low Ki-67, clone MIB-1 LI in a nonfunctioning gonadotroph adenoma of the pituitary. Approx 1% of adenoma cells show nuclear reactivity (ABC 10X).

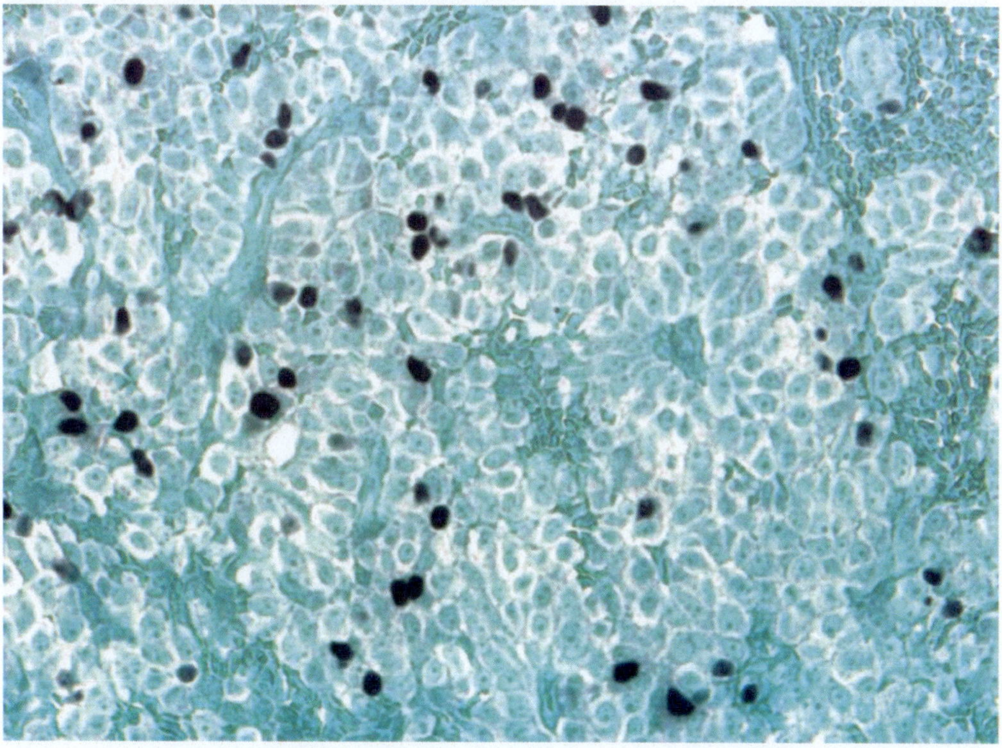

Figure 3. This silent, type 1 corticotroph adenoma shows a 5% Ki-67 LI (ABC 20X).

Gender - Age

Many investigators have not established a significant association between Ki-67 staining and the age at diagnosis or gender in pituitary adenomas (Landolt et al. 1987, Knosp et al. 1989, Shibuya et al. 1992, Abe et al. 1997, Mastronardi et al. 1999, Losa et al. 2000b, Mastronardi et al. 2001, Tanaka et al. 2003, Pizzaro et al. 2004). However, some studies have revealed an inverse correlation of proliferative indices with age (Yonesawa et al. 1997, Losa et al. 2000b); Jaffrain-Rea et al. (2002) also confirmed this finding in functioning adenomas, whereas nonfunctioning pituitary adenomas (NFPA) appeared to be independent of age or gender. Delgrange et al. (1997), in a study of prolactinomas, reported no correlation of age and Ki-67 staining and a predominance of Ki-67 LI in male patients, which was not statistically significant.

Tumor Size

Few studies have demonstrated an association of Ki-67 LI with tumor size (Turner et al. 2000a). Jaffrain-Rea et al. (2002) showed a significant correlation of high Ki-67 LI and the presence of macroadenomas (size > 10mm), particularly with adrenocorticotropin (ACTH) and prolactin (PRL) secreting adenomas, and in adenomas with supra-sellar extension, but not in NFPA. They examined the variability of Ki-67 LI, which tended to increase with the increase of the size of the adenoma. Similar findings were reported by Hsu et al. (1993), with the majority of the tumors examined being macroadenomas with extra-sellar extension. Losa et al. (2000a) demonstrated a significant correlation of Ki-67 LI and poor surgical outcome with maximum diameter of ACTH-secreting adenomas, considering tumor size as the strongest predictor for surgical outcome, although this finding was not confirmed in another study (Losa et al. 2000b). Turner et al. (2000b) reported higher Ki-67 LI in macro-prolactinomas compared with micro-prolactinomas, whereas in the other types of adenomas there was no significant relationship between tumor size and Ki-67 LI. Many other studies have also not found an association between the size of pituitary tumors and Ki-67 LI (Landolt et al. 1987, Knosp et al. 1989, Thapar et al. 1996c, Abe et al. 1997, Delgrange et al. 1997, Mastronardi et al. 1999, Mastronardi et al. 2001, Suliman et al. 2001, Tanaka et al. 2003).

Secretion Status

Regarding the association of Ki-67 LI with the secretory status of pituitary adenomas, many investigators have found no significant correlation of proliferative indices between functioning adenomas and NFPA (Abe et al. 1997, Knosp et al. 1989, Mastronardi et al. 1999, Mastronardi et al. 2001, Pizzaro et al. 2004). However, others have found a strong positive correlation between higher levels of Ki-67 LI and hormone secretion (Landolt et al. 1987, Shibuya et al. 1992, Pegolo et al. 1995, Thapar et al. 1996c). Jaffrain-Rea et al. (2002) reported significant differences of Ki-67 LI and its variations between NFPA and untreated functioning adenomas, with the later exhibiting higher levels of Ki-67 LI, whereas there was no difference between NFPA and pre-treated functioning adenomas, suggesting that preoperative treatment influences significantly the proliferative status of functioning adenomas. Examining the correlation of proliferative rate with the secretory type of pituitary tumors, a great variety of different published data exists. Landolt et al.(1987) reported higher Ki-67 LI in GH secreting adenomas, compared to other types of pituitary tumors with the lowest levels observed in NFPA while ACTH and PRL secreting adenomas had intermediate values. Thapar et al. (1996c) demonstrated highest Ki-67 LI in prolactinomas and lowest in oncocytomas. Other investigators (Asano et al. 1996, Jaffrain-Rea et al. 2002) also found higher levels in prolactinomas, whereas Mastronardi et al. (1999) found significant higher proliferative indices only in ACTH secreting adenomas. Pizzaro et al. (2004), besides a predominance of Ki-67 LI levels in ACTH secreting adenomas, found no significant correlation of the secretory type of the pituitary tumor and the proliferative indices; these findings were later on confirmed by Abe et al. (1997). Pernicone et al. (1996) reported that 30% of pituitary carcinomas are ACTH-secreting tumors, supporting the finding of high proliferation potential in those adenomas.

Growth Rate

An attempt has also been made to assess the growth rate of pituitary tumors by estimating the growth velocity of the tumor, examining the increase of tumor's volume or apoptotic rate through periods of time, and compare them with staining indices. Ekrabullah et al. (1996) estimated tumor volume doubling time (TVDT) by calculating the increase of the tumor volume over a certain period of time, using CT or MRI imaging, in cured and regrowing NFPA. They compared them with Ki-67 LI, demonstrating an inverse correlation of TVDT and Ki-67 LI, which was significantly higher in the recurrent group. Tanaka et al. (2003) estimating TVDT, using the same method as the former investigators, found a positive correlation with age, demonstrating a significant longer TVDT in elderly patients, and an inverse correlation with Ki-67 LI but not with invasion of the cavernous sinuses or with tumor volume. Abe et al. (1997) demonstrated a regrowth rate of 100%, 50% and 16% in adenomas, based on radiological findings, with Ki-67 LI over 3,5%, ≥1,5% and <1,5% respectively. Hoenegger et al. (2003) estimated the percentage of the daily growth, based on CT or MRI imaging studies and calculation of the tumor volume over a certain period of time, in a group of NFPA, demonstrating a significant correlation between high Ki-67 LI and the daily increase of these tumors.

Invasion

Invasive adenomas comprise approximately 35-42% of pituitary adenomas (Scheithauer et al. 1986). The morphology of non-invasive, invasive adenomas and carcinomas is often uniform and without distinguishing characteristics. Many investigators attempted to identify a possible association of proliferative markers with aggressive behavior and invasion, and indicated the dependence of invasion on biological factors, especially when some speculated that invasion maybe due to factors produced by the tumor (Kawamoto et al. 1995, Pizzaro et al. 2004). Most of the studies that have attempted to estimate the invasive potential of pituitary adenomas, are in favor of a positive correlation with the KI-67 LI. The differences that appeared in early studies were due to the different estimation of the degree of invasion. Histological invasion is reported to approach 90% (Selman et al. 1986), whereas invasive behavior assessed radiologicaly or surgically is found in 35% of the adenomas (Scheithauer et al. 1986, Selman et al. 1986). Gross invasion seems more meaningful for establishing a relationship with proliferative markers, as dural invasion is present in even the most indolent adenomas, and the use of Magnetic Resonance Imaging (MRI) instead of computed tomography (CT) coincides with the surgeon's impression during surgery and can be accurately used (Thapar et al. 1996c, Blevins et al. 1998, Losa et al. 2000b, Mastronardi et al. 2001).

Studies in the late 1980s demonstrated a significant correlation of high Ki-67 LI obtained in frozen sections with the histological invasion of pituitary tumors (Landolt et al. 1987, Knosp et al. 1989); radiologicaly, invasive tumors also exhibited higher Ki-67 LI although this was not statistically significant. Several reports over the following years, using Ki-67 MIB-1 antibody in formalin-fixed paraffin sections confirmed the positive association of higher MIB-1 LI and the invasive potential, estimating invasion radiologically or by surgeon's impression during operation of pituitary tumors (Buchfelder et al. 1996, Blevins et al. 1998, Mastronardi et al. 1999, Zao et al. 1999, Mastronardi et al. 2001, Suliman et al. 2001, Jaffrain-Rea et al. 2002, Pizzaro et al. 2004) or estimating invasion by histology (Selman et al. 1986, Daita and Yonemasu 1996). In one study (Thapar et al. 1996c) malignant and invasive tumors appeared to have much higher Ki-67 LI compared to non-invasive adenomas, 11.9% vs. 4.66% vs. 1.37% respectively. Some of them reported a significant positive correlation when invasion of the cavernous sinuses was considered (Mastronardi et al. 1999, Mastronardi et al. 2001, Jaffrain-Rea et al. 2002). Other authors have also reported higher levels of MIB-1 LI in invasive tumors, although no statistically significant differences were found (Atkin et al. 1997, Delgrange et al. 1997). Several other studies have also failed to document a correlation between MIB-1 LI and tumor invasiveness assessed by histology (Kawamoto et al. 1995, Gardour-Edwards et al. 1995, Pegolo et al. 1995, Yonesawa et al. 1997, Abe et al. 1997, Losa et al. 2000b, Yokoyama et al. 2001, Tanaka et al. 2003, Honegger et al. 2003). However, there was considerable variation of the examined material, as different types (Delgrange et al. 1997, Losa et al. 2000b, Tanaka et al. 2003, Honegger et al. 2003) or mixed population of pituitary adenomas have been studied (Gardour-Edwards et al. 1995, Thapar et al. 1996c, Atkin et al. 1997, Abe et al. 1997, Mastronardi et al. 1999, Mastronardi et al. 2001). Jaffrain-Rea et al. (2002) found significant higher proliferative rates in functioning invasive adenomas, especially when infiltration of cavernous sinuses was present or no pre-operative treatment was applied.

Recurrence

A great proportion of pituitary adenomas exhibits locally aggressive behavior, infiltrating surrounding tissues, therefore minimizing the likelihood of complete surgical resection. The regrowth of a previously resected pituitary tumor remains always a possibility if there is residual tumor, even if it exhibits low values of proliferative indices. Losa et al. (2000b) reported a relapse rate of 33.8% in NFPA after 28.6 ± 4.8 months from the time of surgery, in the group of patients with residual disease. The presence of any relationship between Ki-67 LI and tumor recurrence could help to distinguish a slow growing from a rapid growing tumor, therefore selecting patients in whom a closer follow-up with or without adjuvant therapy is required. Although a number of reports have found no correlation between proliferating indices, such as Ki-67 and the possibility of local recurrence (Yonesawa et al. 1997, Losa et al. 2000a, Losa et al. 2000b, Pizzaro et al. 2004), others have demonstrated a significant positive correlation of this proliferative marker and tumor recurrence (Shiduya et al. 1992, Ekrabullah et al. 1996, Abe et al. 1997, Mizoue et al. 1997). This positive association was not present in all types of pituitary tumors but occurred in only some types of pituitary tumors, as in a study of Jaffrain-Rea et al. (2002), where this finding appeared only in functioning untreated adenomas. Nakabayashi et al. (2001) found a significant association of cyclin A and tumor recurrence and also a linear correlation of cyclin A and Ki-67 LI, especially in macroadenomas, suggesting that these factors and subtotal surgical resection maybe highly significant for the prediction of remission. Very high values of Ki-67 LI may help identify the subset of tumors with highly aggressive behavior, prevailing their ability to metastasize.

The difficulty in establishing a cut off value of Ki-67 LI capable to distinguish invasive tumors designated to develop a benign behavior from the aggressive ones is due to the overlap of Ki-67 values that occurs in these two entities. Several studies have attempted to calculate a clear threshold that could identify the great majority of pituitary adenomas designated to develop a more aggressive tumor behavior. Jaffrain-rea et al. (2002) suggested a Ki-67 LI threshold of 2.5% for NFPA or previously treated functioning adenomas and a 6% LI for untreated functioning adenomas. Abe et al. (1997) exhibited an LI value of 3.5% for adenomas that had a regrowth rate of 100% and the higher likelihood to regrow (50% regrowth rate) when LI is over 1.5%. Two other studies confirmed the value of 1.5% as being the cut off value with the greatest risk of rapid regrowth (Shibuya et al. 1992, Hoenegger et al. 2003). Mastronardi et al. (1999) suggested a threshold value of 3.5% for invasive adenomas and 5% for adenomas exhibiting invasion into the cavernous sinuses. In addition, a system for grading invasion was proposed in relation to Ki-67 LI (grade 0: non-invasive adenomas with a mean LI of 2%, grade I: invasive adenomas with a mean Ki-67 LI of 3.7%, grade II: adenomas infiltrating the cavernous sinuses and exhibiting a mean Ki-67 LI of 5.6%, grade III: pituitary carcinoma with Ki-67 LI of 36%). Pizzaro et al. (2004) failed to show a clear cut off value of proliferative indices that could identify aggressive adenomas, despite the significantly higher Ki-67 LI values obtained in invasive adenomas due to considerable overlap with the values obtained from patients with non-invasive adenomas. Thapar et al. (1996c) suggested that a 3% value could distinguish invasive from non-invasive pituitary tumors, with sensitivity and specificity of 72.7% and 97.3%, respectively; the positive predictive value was 96% and the negative predictive value was 80%. The growth fraction in all these studies seems to reflect a feature of more rapidly growing adenomas, although it is not justified to use Ki-67 LI alone to predict the biological behavior of pituitary tumors.

Preoperative Treatment

Delgrange et al. 1997 reported a strong correlation between the administration of preoperative treatment, i.e. dopamine agonists, and tumor size in a study of 92 prolactinomas, but no correlation with proliferative indices in treated and untreated adenomas. Treatment-resistant tumors exhibited higher Ki-67 LI, particularly, in male patients. In a study of Mastronardi et al. (1999), preoperative treatment with bromocriptine showed no effect on Ki-67 LI of prolactinomas or mixed adenomas with predominant prolactin expression, whereas Jaffrain-Rea et al. (2002) reported lower Ki-67 LI following treatment of adenomas secreting GH or PRL.

Carcinomas

Relatively few studies have enclosed pituitary carcinomas in their investigation material, as these tumors are particularly rare. In many occasions their behavior is indistinguishable from the much more common benign adenomas except that the clinical course is punctuated with multiple recurrences and the development of metastases. Despite the reported high levels of Ki-67 LI (Thapar et al. 1996c), “paradoxically'' low levels can also be observed particularly at first surgery (Pernicone et al. 1997), suggesting that these tumors arise from benign proliferations secondary to de novo molecular events (Karga et al. 1992). In a study of Thapar et al. (1996c) the carcinomas presented the highest growth fractions as assessed by Ki67 Li (mean 11.91%), but with a wide range of LIs (0%-21.9%), suggesting that growth rate is not the primary determinant of the metastatic capability. Low Ki-67 LI in pituitary carcinomas may be attributed to delayed tissue fixation or suppression of proliferation by preoperative medical treatment (Cross et al. 1990). Nevertheless, as the majority of invasive tumors exhibit Ki-67 LI values less than 10%, LI over 10% should always raise suspicion about the malignant potential of the tumor (Thapar et al. 1996c, Pernicone et al. 1997, Gaffey et al. 2002, Kaltsas et al. 2005).

Correlation with other Parameters

Studying the relationship of Ki-67 staining with previous techniques used for the assessment of tumor proliferative state, a significant but weak linear correlation with the number of mitoses has been reported (Landolt et al. 1987, Thapar et al. 1996a). Jaffrain-Rea et al. (2002) confirmed this association in functioning pituitary adenomas and demonstrated a reduction of mitoses when pre-operative treatment was applied; however, others have found no correlation (Gardour-Edwards et al. 1995). In addition, a significant correlation of Ki-67 LI and BrdU LI was found (Nagashima et al. 1986, Sasaki et al. 1988, Girino et al. 1990, Shibuya et al. 1992, Ikeda et al. 1992, Birner et al. 2001, Muskelishvilli et al. 2003) and also a strong association between p53 staining and Ki-67, clone MIB-1 LI (Thapar et al. 1996b, Suliman et al. 2001). Studying the possible correlation of Ki-67 with cyclins, a significant relationship of Ki-67 LI and cyclin D, but not cyclins A,B,E, was reported by Turner et al.

(2000a), although another study showed a linear correlation of KI-67 and cyclin A (Nakabayashi et al. 2001). Comparing PCNA LI and Ki-67 LI, a significant association has been reported (Atkin et al. 1997) in vitro, although higher levels of Ki-67 LI were found in vivo, probably due to the slow decrease of the antigen in quiescent cells. Ekrabullah et al. (1996) reported differences of PCNA LI and Ki-67, clone MIB-1 LI between cured and recurrent adenomas. In another study, Turner et al. (2000b) exhibited a lack of association between Ki-67 LI and angiogenesis, probably due to the fact that angiogenesis expresses the speed of progression through the cell cycle, whereas Ki-67 LI measures the proportion of the cells entered the cell cycle. Shibuya et al. (1992) found a significant correlation between Ki-67 LI and DNA polymerase α staining, with differences of both labeling indices among pituitary adenoma subtypes and Saeger et al. (2001) reported a positive correlation of Topoisomerase IIα with Ki-67, clone MIB-1 LI; however, another study (Maier et al. 1990) failed to correlate Ki-67 LI with the mean number of Ag-NORs. Investigating apoptosis, Losa et al. (2000a) determined the mean apoptotic index and Ki-67 LI in a group of ACTH producing adenomas with a significant correlation between them.

Original Results

Table 1. Analysis of Ki-67 in 73 pituitary adenomas/correlation with clinical-hormonal-morphological features

Gender	**Number (Frequencies)**	**Mean Ki-67 LI ± Standard error of mean**	**p**
Male	40 (54.8%)	1.51% (± 0.25%) (range 0.5-10%)	
Female	33 (45.2%)	2.24% (± 0.89%) (range 0.5-30%)	p: 0.968 (>0.05)
Total	*73* (100%)		
Mean age 50yrs(range 23-76)			
Size			
Macroadenomas*	66 (90.4%)	1.87% (± 0.46%) (range 0.5-30%)	
Microadenomas	7 (9.6%)	1.57% (± 0.63%) (range 0.5-5%)	p: 0.799 (>0.05)
Function			
Functioning PA	36 (49.3%)	1,33% (± 0.19%)(range 0.5-5%)	
Non-functioning PA	37 (50.7%)	2,33% (± 0.79%)(range 0.5-30%)	p: 0.299 (>0.05)
Type			
NFPA	37 (50.7%)	2.34% (± 0.815%) (range 0.5-30%)	
ACTH	6 (8.2%)	1.5% (± 0.74%) (range 0.5-5%)	
GH	27 (37%)	1.33% (± 0.19%) (range 0.5-3.5%)	
PRL	3 (4.1%)	1.0% (± 0.5%) (range 0.5-2%)	p: 0.68 (>0.05)
Invasion**			
Non-invasive PA	15 (20.5%)	1.4% (± 0.33%) (range 0.5-5%)	
Invasive PA	58 (79.5%)	1.95% (± 0.52%) (range 0.5-30%)	p: 0.653 (>0.05)

Table 1 (Continued)

Invasion CS	Number (Frequencies)	Mean Ki-67 LI ± Standard error of mean	p
Non-invasive PA	15 (20.5%)	1.4% (± 0.33%) (range 0.5-5%)	
Invasion in CS	26 (35.7%)	2.78% (± 1.15%) (range 0.5-30%)	
Invasion but not in CS	32 (43.8%)	1.28% (± 0.93%) (range 0.5-4.5%)	p: 0.441 (>0.05)
Non-invasive PA	15(20.5%)	1.4% (± 0.33%) (range 0.5-5%)	
Invasion in one region	28 (38.4%)	1.05% (± 0.118%) (range 0.5-2.5%)	
Invasion in more than one regions	30 (41.1%)	2.8 % (± 0.998%) (range 0.5-30%)	p: 0.044 (p<0.05)

[†] Pituitary adenomas
[*] Microadenomas > 10mm
Macroadenomas ≤ 10mm
[***] Hardy's classification
[††] CS: Cavernous sinuses

Seventy-three patients (40 males), mean age 50 yrs (range 23-76 yrs), with pituitary tumors histologically proved to be adenomas underwent a transphenoidal resection in our hospital from 1998 to 2004. Ki-67 LI of the tumor was performed using the MIB-1 epitope. Similarly to others we investigated the presence of a possible correlation between the size and the secretory potential of the adenoma and its invasiveness with the Ki-67 LI. Tumor invasiveness was assessed by MRI using Hardy's (Hardy 1973) classification to denote invasiveness. Sixty-six patients had macroadenomas (>10mm) and 7 microadenomas (≤10mm). Invasion was present in 58 (79.5 %) adenomas (23 suprasellar, 3 cavernous sinuses, 2 sphenoid sinus), whereas 15 (20.5 %) adenomas were noninvasive, intrasellar. Amongst the invasive adenomas more than 30 exhibited invasion in one region. Thirty-seven were NFPA and thirty-six were functioning adenomas (6 corticotroph, 27 somatotroph adenomas and 3 prolactinomas). Statistical analysis was performed using the two-sample Mann-Whitney U-test and the results are tabulated in Table 1. Although higher levels of Ki-67 LI were obtained in NFPA compared to functioning adenomas, no statistically significant differences were found. The mean Ki-67 LI of NFPA and functioning adenomas was 2.33% ± 0.8% (range 0.5%-30%) and 1.33% ± 0.19% (range 0.5%-5%) (mean ± standard error of mean) respectively (p>0.05). Macroadenomas presented a slightly higher Ki-67 LI from that of microadenomas. The mean Ki-67 LI was 1.87% ± 0.46% (range 0.5%-30%) in macroadenomas and 1.57% ± 0.6% (range 0.5%-5%) in microadenomas (p>0.05).

Invasive tumors had higher levels of LI than non-invasive, particularly the ones infiltrating the cavernous sinuses and the ones infiltrating more than one region around the sella turnica; however, only the later exhibited statistical significance. The mean Ki-67 LI of noninvasive and invasive tumors was 1.4% ± 0.33% (range 0.5%-5%) and 1.95% ± 0.53% (range 0.5%-30%) respectively. Adenomas with evidence of invasion in more than one regions (n=30) exhibited mean Ki-67 LI 2.8% ± 0.99% (range 0.5%-30%) compared to adenomas with no invasion and tumors with invasion in only one region (p<0.05). Invasion of cavernous sinuses exhibited Ki-67 LI 2.78% ± 1.15% (range 0.5%-30%), whereas invasion of other regions had an LI of 1.28% ± 0.165% (range 0.5%-4.5%). In addition, estimating Ki-

67 LI > 3% in our material, no significant relation was found to the tumor size, invation or function (Table 2).

Table 2. Adenomas exhibiting Ki-67 LI >3%

	Total Number	N (Frequency)	p
Microadenomas	7	1 (14.3%)	
Macroadenomas	66	4 (6%)	p>0.05
Non-invasive PA	15	1 (6.7%)	
Invasive PA	58	4(6.9%)	p>0.05
Non-functioning PA	37	2 (5.6%)	
Functioning PA	36	3 (8.1%)	p>0.05
NFPA	37	3 (8.1%)	
ACTH	6	1 (16.7%)	
GH	27	1 (3.7%)	
PRL	3	0 (0%)	p>0.

*Pituitary adenomas

Previous analysis using the Kolmogorov-Smirnov test did not show statistical difference in adenomas invading more than one regions (Stathopoulou et al. 2005).

The discrepancies observed between our data and those reported by other investigators may be attributed to the wide range of Ki-67 LI values, even in NFPA, and the small number of the adenomas examined, especially of prolactinomas.

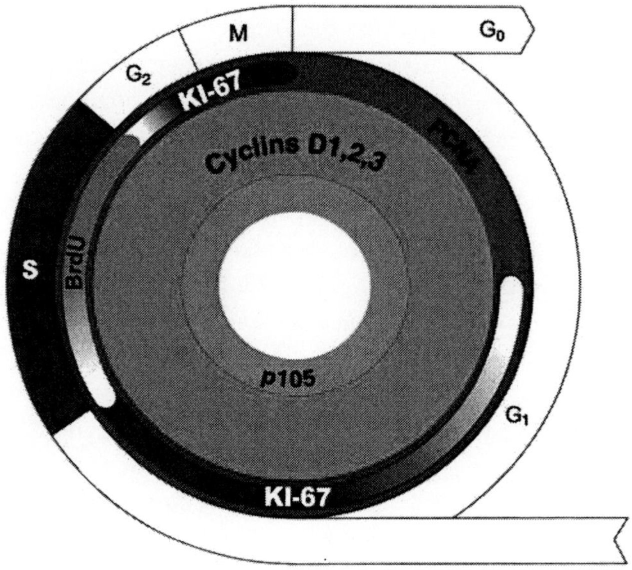

Figure 4. The presence of specific molecules during the phases of cell cycle

Comment

Pituitary adenomas, although in their majority are slow growing benign tumors, they can occasionally exhibit rapid growth, infiltrating surrounding tissues and producing neurological symptoms of an intracranial mass. This sequence of events is apart of the symptoms that appear from the increased hormone levels in the case of functioning adenomas. Morphological features, such as nuclear pleomorphism, cytological atypia, high cellularity and brisk mitotic activity, although in most tumor models correlate with aggressive behavior, have limited use in assessing invasiveness, recurrence potential, and the biologic behavior of pituitary adenomas. As many adenomas are already invasive by the time of diagnosis, a complete surgical excision is not possible and recurrence may be only regrowth of the residual tumor. A potential mean of predicting tumoral behavior may be the assessment of cell proliferation by measuring the proportion of cells entering the cell cycle. The results of many studies investigating cell kinetics, have revealed several discrepancies of the means used to assess the cells being in the S-phase fraction, and thus estimate the growth potential of pituitary adenomas, which are generally slow growing tumors (Nagashima et al. 1986). In addition, no general correlations appear between DNA and the morphologic growth pattern and/or criteria of malignancy (Anniko et al. 1984). Refined morphological methods, such as ultrastructual morphometry and electron microscopy, are not routinely applicable in determining growth characteristics (Ludecke et al. 1985). The investigation of specific molecules that participate in cell proliferation (Figure 4) with the use of monoclonal antibodies has served as a mean to distinguish tumors with a more indolent profile from those with aggressive potential. However, more knowledge is required regarding the role of cyclins, inhibitors of cell cycle, factors controlling apoptosis and other genetic changes to assess the growth potential of pituitary adenomas (Turner and Wass 1999, Suhardja et al. 2001, Ironside et al. 2003) Several studies have investigated the role of local factors and/or proteolytic enzymes or other regulators and other unknown mechanisms, bearing upon invasive potential of pituitary adenomas and perhaps regulating components of extracellular matrix, independent of the proliferative potential of the tumors (Alvaro et al. 1993). Amongst them, estimation of Ki-67 LI seems to be the most promising (Saeger 2004), currently available, marker of assessing the proliferation potential of pituitary tumors. According to the recent World Health Organization classification of endocrine neoplasms, an increased Ki-67 LI (>3%) is a strong predictive factor for adenomas with aggressive potential. In combination with high mitotic activity and/or the presence of extensive p53 immunoreactivity such adenomas should be termed "atypical" (Figure 5), to denote their potential aggressive profile and the possibility of future malignant transformation (Lloyd et al. 2004). Some authors propose the term "atypical" for adenomas showing Ki-67 LI more that 10% irrespective p53 immunoreactivity (Kaltsas et al. 2005).

Conclusion

Estimating the growth fraction is not sufficient alone to predict pituitary tumor growth, as it relates to the number of proliferating cells and not to the time needed to complete the cell cycle. As it reflects the state and not the rate of proliferation and since it is only one factor influencing tumor behavior, this parameter alone cannot predict but rather provide the clinician with prognostic information. As Ki-67 LI is the most reliable marker of proliferative potential in pituitary adenomas to date, high values, especially over 3%, should alert the clinician for a more aggressive potential and a close follow up of the particular tumor. It can also be used as an indicator of the tumors that may need further treatment with adjuvant medical therapy and/or radiotherapy. Many other factors, local or not, remain to be investigated, in an attempt to understand the unknown mechanisms that lead a benign pituitary adenoma to express a more aggressive profile and maybe to undergo malignant transformation.

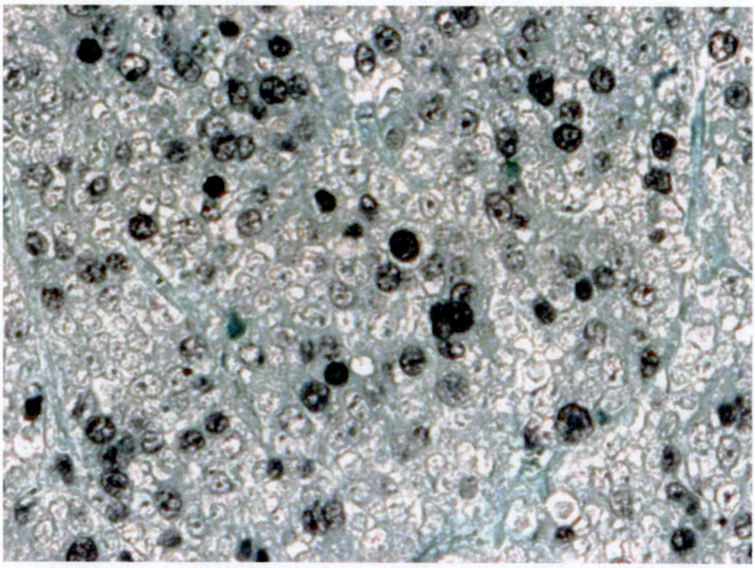

Figure 5. Extensive immunoreactivity for p53. Note strong nuclear staining in several cells in this functioning corticotroph adenoma designated "atypical" (ABC 40X).

References

Abe, T., Sanno, N., Osamura, Y. R. and Matsumoto, K. (1997). Proliferative potential in Pituitary adenomas: Measurement by monoclonal antibody MIB-1. *Acta Neurochir* (Wien), 139, 613-618.

Ahyai, A., Hori, A., Bockermann, V., Rama, B., Blech, M. and Markakis, E. (1988). Impulse cytophotometric DNA analysis in pituitary adenomas. *Neurosurg Rev,* 11, 77-86.

Alvaro, V., Levy, L., Dubray, C., Roche, A., Peillon, F., Quetrat, B. and Joubert, D. (1993). Invasive human pituitary tumors express a point-mutated alpha-protein kinase-C. *J Clin Endocrinol Metab,* 77, 1125-1129.

Anniko, M., Tribukait, B. and Wersall, J. (1983). The significance of a high percentage of S-phase cells in human pituitary tumors. *ORL J Otorhinolaryngol Relat Spec,* 45, 177-186.

Anniko, M., Holm, L. E., Tribukait, B. and Wersall, J. (1981). Aneuploid DNA pattern in human pituitary adenomas. *Arch Otorhinolaryngol,* 230, 1-4.

Anniko, M., Tribukait, B. and Wersall, J. (1984). DNA ploidy and cell phase in human pituitary tumors. *Cancer,* 53, 1708-1713.

Asa, S. and Ezzat, S. (1988). The cytogenesis and pathogenesis of pituitary adenomas. *Endocr Rev,* 19, 798-827.

Asano, K., Kubo, O., Tajika, Y., Huang, M. C. and Takamura, K. (1996). The relationship between cell proliferation and secretory activity in pituitary adenomas. A review of 63 cases. *No To Shinkei,* 48, 543-549.

Atkin, L. S., Green, L. V., Hipkin, J. L., Landolt, M. A., Foy, M. P., Jeffreys, V. R. and White, C. M. (1997). A comparison of proliferation indices in human anterior pituitary adenomas using formalin-fixed tissue and in vitro cell culture. *J Neurosurg,* 87, 85-88.

Atkin, N. B. and Kay, B. (1979). Prognostic significance of modal DNA value and other factors in malignant tumors, based in 1465 cases. *Brit J Cancer,* 40, 210-221.

Auer, G., Caspersson, T. and Wallgren, A. (1980). DNA content and survival in mammary carcinoma. *Anal Quant Cytol,* 3, 161-165.

Bamberger, C.M., Fehn, M., Bamberger, A. M., Ludecke, D. K., Beil, F. U., Saeger, W. and Schulte, H. M. (1999). Reduced expression levels of the cell-cycle inhibitor p27Kip1 in human pituitary adenomas. *Eur J Endocr,* 140, 250-255.

Birner, P., Ritzi, M., Musahl, C., Knippers, R., Gerdes, J., Voigtlander, T., Budka, H. and Hainfellner, J. (2001). Immunohistochemical detection of cell growth fraction in formalin-fixed and paraffin-embedded murine tissue. *Am J Pathol,* 158, 1991-1996.

Blevins, L. S. Jr., Verity, D. K. and Allen, G. (1998). Aggressive pituitary tumors. *Oncology,* 12, 1307-1312. Discussion. 1315-1318

Braun, N., Papadopoulos, T. and Muller-Hermelink, H. K. (1988). Cell cycle dependent distribution of the proliferation-associated Ki-67 antigen in human embryonic lung cells. *Virchows Arch B Cell Pathol Incl Mol Pathol,* 56, 25-33.

Brown, D.C. and Gatter, K.C. (1990). Monoclonal antibody Ki-67: its use in histopathology. *Histopathol,* 17, 489-503.

Bruno, S. and Darzynkiewicz, Z. (1992). Cell cycle dependent expression and stability of the nuclear protein detected by Ki-67 antibody in HL-60 cells. *Cell Prolif,* 25, 31-40.

Buchfelder, M., Fahlbusch, R., Adams, E. F., Kiesewetter, F. and Thierauf, P. (1996). Proliferation parameters for pituitary adenomas. *Acta Neurochir Suppl,* 65, 18-21.

Buckley, N., Bates, A. S., Broome, J. C., Strange, R.C., Perrett, C. W., Burke, C. W. and Clayton, R. N. (1994). P53 protein accumulates in Cushings adenomas and invasive non-functional adenomas. *J Clin Endocr Metabol,* 79, 1513-1516.

Chatterjee, S., May, P., Forster, G., Spiller, D. and Jeffreys, R. (1993). Prediction of recurrence in pituitary tumors: a flow cytometric study using in vivo bromodeoxyuridine. *Brit J Neurosurg,* 7, 165-170.

Cho, K. G., Nagashima, T., Barnwell, S. and Hoshino, T. (1988). Flow cytometric determination of modal DNA population in relation to proliferative potential of human intracranial tumors. *J Neurosurg,* 69, 588-592.

Ciric, I., Mikhael, M. and Stafford, T. (1983). Transphenoidal microsurgery of pituitary adenomas. *Int J Radiat Oncol Biol Phys,* 15, 305-309.

Clayton, R. N., Pfeifer, M., Atkinson, A. B., Belchetz, P., Wass, J. A. H., Kyrodimou, E., Vanderpump, M., Simpson, D., Bicknell, J. and Farrell, W. (2000). Different patterns of allelic loss (loss of heterozygosity) in recurrent human pituitary tumors provide evidence for multiclonal origins. *Clin Cancer Res,* 6, 3973-3982.

Cross, S. S., Start, R. D. and Smith, J. H. (1990). Does delay in fixation affect the number of mitotic figures in processed tissue? *J Clin Pathol,* 43, 597-599.

Cunningham, J., Lust, J. A., Schaid, D. J., Bren, G. D., Carpenter, H. A., Rizza, E., Kovach, J. S. and Thibodeau, S. N. (1992). Expression of p53 and 17p allelic loss in colorectal carcinoma. *Cancer Res,* 52, 1974-1980.

Daita, G. and Yonemasu, Y. (1996). Dural invasion and proliferative potential of pituitary adenomas. *Neurol Med Chir,* 36, 211-214.

Delgrange, E., Trouillas, J., Maiter, D., Donckier, J. and Tourniaire, J. (1997). Sex-related difference in the growth of prolactinomas: A clinical and proliferation marker study. *J Clin Endocr Metabol,* 82, 2102-2107.

Denton, T. E., Brook, W. R. and Howell, W. M. (1977). A technique for the simultaneous staining of both nucleolar organizer regions and kinetochores of human chromosomes with silver. *Stain Technol,* 52, 311-313.

Ebersold, M. J., Quast, L. M. and Laws, E. R. Jr. (1986). Long-term results in transphenoidal removal of nonfunctioning pituitary adenomas. *J Neurosurg,* 64, 713-719.

Ekrabullah, S.M., Saitoh, Y., Arita, N., Ohnishi, T. and Hayakawa, T. (1996). The correlation of Ki-67 staining indices in tumor doubling times in regrowing non-functioning adenomas. *Acta Neurochir* (Wien), 138, 1449-1455.

Fitzgibbons, P. L., Appley, A., Turner, R. R., Bishop, P., Parker, J., Breeze, R., Weiss, M. and Apuzzo, J. (1988). Flow Cytometric Analysis of pituitary tumors. *Cancer,* 62,1556-1560.

Frederickson, P., Reske-Nielsen, E. and Bichel, P. (1978). Flow cytometry in tumors of the brain. *Acta Neuropathol* (Berl), 41, 179-183.

Gaffey, T. A., Scheithauer, B. W., Loyd, R. V., Burger, P. C., Robbins, P , Fereidooni, F., Hotvath, E., Kovacs, K., Kuroki, T., Young, W. F., Sebo, T. J., Riehl, D. L. and Belzeberg, A. J. (2002). Corticotroph carcinoma of the pituitary : a clinicopathological study. *J Neurosurg,* 96, 352-360.

Galand, P. and Degraef, C. (1989). Cyclin/PCNA immunostaining as an alternative to titriated thymidine pulse labeling for marking S-phase cells in paraffin sections and human tissues. *Cell Tissue Kinet,* 22, 383-392.

Garcia, R. L., Coltera, M. D. and Gown, A. M. (1989). Analysis of proliferative grade using anti-PCNA/cyclin monoclonal antibodies in fixed, embedded tissues. Comparison with flow cytometric analysis. *Am J Pathol,* 134, 733-739.

Gardour-Edwards, R., Kapadia, B. S., Janecka, P. I., Martinez, J. and Barnes, L. (1995). Biologic markers of invasive pituitary adenomas involving the sphenoid sinus. *Mod Pathol,* 8, 160-164.

Gattoretti, G., Becker, M.H.G., Key, G., Duchrow, M., Schlüter, C., Galle, J. and Gerdes, J. (1992). Monoclonal antibodies against recombinant parts of the Ki-67 antigen (MIB-1 and MIB-3) detect proliferating cells in microwave – processed formalin-fixed paraffin sections. *J Pathol,* 168, 357-363.

Gerdes, J., Becker, M. H. G. and Key, G.(1992). Immunohistological detection of tumor growth fraction (Ki-67 antigen) in formalin-fixed and routinely processed tissues. *J Pathol,* 168, 85-87.

Gerdes, J., Lemke, H., Baisch, H., Wacker, H. H., Schab, U. and Stein, H. (1984). Cell cycle analysis of a cell proliferation-associated human nuclear antigen defined by the monoclonal antibody Ki-67. *J Immunol,* 133, 1710-1715.

Gerdes, J., Schab, U., Lemke, H. and Stein, H. (1983). Production of a mouse monoclonal antibody reactive with a human nuclear antigen associated with cell proliferation. *Int. J. Cancer,* 31, 13-20.

Girino, M., Riccardi, A., Danova, M., Gaetani, P., Butti, G., Giordanno, M. and Cuomo, A. (1990). Immunocytochemical evaluation of proliferative activity in human brain tumors. *Anal Cell Pathol,* 2, 269-275.

Gratzner, H. G. (1982). Monoclonal antibody to 5-bromo- and 5-iododeoxyuridine: a new reagent for detection of DNA replication. *Science,* 218, 474-476.

Hall, P. A., Levinson, D. A., Woods, A. L., Yu, C. C., Kellock, D. B., Watkins, J. A., Barnes, D. M., Gillett, C. E., Camplejohn, R., Dover, R., Waseem, N. H. and Lane, D. P. (1990). Proliferating cell nuclear antigen (PCNA) immunolocalization in paraffin sections: an index of cell proliferation with evidence of deregulated expression in some neoplasms. *J Pathol,* 162, 285-294.

Harada, K., Arita, K., Kurisu, K., and Tahara, H.(2000). Telomerase activity and the expression of telomerase components in pituitary adenoma with malignant transformation. *Surg Neurol,* 53, 267-274.

Hardy, J. (1973). Transphenoidal surgery of hypersecreting pituitary tumors. In: Diagnosis and treatment of pituitary tumors. PO Kohler, GT Ross, Eds. *Excepta Medica, American Elsevier,* 179-194.

Herman, V., Fragin, J., Gonsky, R., Kovacs, K. and Melmed, S. (1990). Clonal origin of pituitary adenomas. *J Clin Endocrinol Metab,* 71, 1427-1433.

Hockenbery, D., Nuñez, G., Milliman, C., Schreider, R. D. and Korsmeyer, S. J. (1990). Bcl-2 is an inner mitochondrial membrane protein that blocks programmed cell death. *Nature,* 348, 334-336.

Hollstein, M., Rice, K., Greenblatt, M. S., Soussi, T., Fuchs, R., Sorlie, T., Hoving, E., Smith-Sorensen, B., Montesano, R. and Harris, C. C. (1994). Data base of p53 gene somatic mutations in human tumors and cell lines. *Nucleic Acids Res,* 22, 3551-3555.

Honegger, J., Prettin, C., Feuerhake, F., Petrick, M., Schulte-Mönting, J. and Reincke, M. (2003). Expression of Ki-67 antigen in non-functioning pituitary adenomas: Correlation with growth velocity and invasiveness. *J Neurosurg,* 99, 674-679.

Hoshino, T., Nagashima, T., Murovic, J., Wilson, C., Edwards, M., Gutin, P., Davis, R. and DeArmond, S. (1986a). In situ cell kinetics studies on human neuroectodermal tumors with bromodeoxyuridine labeling. *J Neurosurg,* 64, 453-459.

Hoshino, T., Nagashima, T., Cho, K. G., Murovic, J. A., Hodes, J. E., Wilson, C. B., Edwards, M. S. and Pitts, L. H. (1986b). S-phase fraction of human brain tumors in situ measured by uptake of bromodeoxyuridine. *Int J Cancer,* 38, 369-374.

Hsu, D., Hakim, F., Biller, B. M., De La Monte, S., Zervas, N., Klibanski, A. and Hedley-Whyte, T. (1993). Significance of proliferating cell nuclear antigen index in predicting pituitary adenoma recurrence. *J Neurosurg,* 78, 753-761.

Hulting, A. L., Tribukait, B., Bergstrand, G. and Werner, S. (1985). DNA and S-phase representation in human growth hormone producing pituitary adenomas. *Acta Endocrinol* (Copenh), 109, 295-303.

Hulting, A. L., Askensten, U., Tribukait, B., Wersall, J., Auer, G., Grimelius, L., Falkmer, S. and Werner, S. (1989). DNA evaluation in growth hormone producing pituitary adenomas: flow cytometry versus single cell analysis. *Acta Endocrinologica* (Copenh), 121, 317-321.

Ikeda, H. and Yoshimoto, T. (1992). The relationship between c-myc protein expression, the bromodeoxyuridine labeling index and the biological behavior of pituitary adenomas. *Acta Neuropathol* (Berl), 83, 361-364.

Ironside, J. W. (2003). Pituitary gland pathology. *J Clin Pathol,* 56, 561-568.

Jaffrain-Rea, M. L., Di Stefano, D., Minniti, G., Esposito, V., Bultrini, A., Ferretti, E., Santoro, A., Faticanti Scucchi, L., Gulino, A. and Cantore, G. (2002). A critical reappraisal of MIB-1 labelling index significance in a large series of pituitary tumors: secreting versus non-secreting adenomas. *Endocr Rel Cancer,* 9, 103-113.

Jordan, S., Lidhar, K., Korbonits, M., Lowe, D. G. and Grossman, A. (2000). Cyclin D and cyclin E expression in normal and adenomatous pituitary. *Eur J Endocrinol,* 143, R1-R6.

Kaltsas, G., Nomikos, P., Kontogeorgos, G., Buchfelder, M. and Grossman, A. (2005). Diagnosis and management of pituitary carcinomas. *J Clin Endocrinol Metab,* 90, 3089-3099.

Karga, H. J., Alexander, J. M., Hadley-White, E. T., Klibanski, A. and Jameson, J. L. (1992). Ras mutations in human pituitary tumors. *J Clin Endocrinol Metab,* 83, 914-919.

Kawamoto, H., Uozumi, T., Arita, K., Yano, T. and Hirohata, T. (1995). Analysis of the growth rate and cavernous sinus invasion of pituitary adenomas. *Acta Neurochir* (Wien), 136, 37-43.

Keszthelyi, R. et al. Immunomorphological assessment of the new Ki-67 specific rabbit monoclonal SP6 antibody on fixed-embedded tissue sections. Lab vision Corporation datafile.

Keyomarsi, K., O'Leary, N. and Molnar, G. (1994). Cyclin E: a potential prognostic marker for breast cancer. *Cancer Research,* 54, 380-385.

Knosp, E., Kitz, K. and Perneczky, A. (1989). Proliferation Activity in Pituitary adenomas : measurement by monoclonal antibody Ki-67. *Neurosurg,* 25, 927-930.

Knowlton, K., Mancini, M., Creason, S., Morales, C., Hockenbery, D. and Anderson, B. O. (1998). Bcl-2 slows in vitro breast cancer despite its antiapoptotic effect. *J Surg Res,* 76, 22-26.

Kontogeorgos, G., Kapranos, N., Orphanidis, G., Rologis, D. and Kokka, E. (1999a). Molecular cytogenetics of chromosome 11 in pituitary adenomas: a comparison of fluorescence in situ hybridization and DNA ploidy study. *Hum Pathol,* 3, 1377-1382.

Kontogeorgos, G., Kapranos, N., Rologis, D., Vamvassakis, E. and Papadopoulos, N. (1996). DNA measurement in pituitary adenomas – Assessed on imprints by image analysis. *Anal Quant Cytol Histol,* 18, 144-150.

Kontogeorgos, G., Kapranos, N., Thodou, E., Sambaziotis, D. and Tsagarakis, S. (1999b). Immunohistochemical accumulation of p53 in corticotroph adenomas: Relationship with heat shock proteins and apoptosis. *Pituitary,* 1, 207-212.

Korbonits, M., Chahal, H. S., Kaltsas, G., Jordan, S., Urmanova, Y., Khalimova, Z., Harris, P. E., Farrell, W. E., Claret, F. X. and Grossman, A. B. (2002). Expression of phosphorylated p27 (kip1) protein and Jun activation domain- binding protein 1 in human pituitary tumors. *J Clin Endocrinol Metab,* 87, 2635-2643.

Kovacs, K. and Horvath, E. (1986). Tumors of pituitary gland. *Atlas of tumor pathology,* 2nd series, fascicle 21. Bethesda: Armed Forces Institute of Pathology.

Kovacs, K. (1984). Light and electron microscopic pathology of pituitary tumors: Immunohistochemistry. In: Black PMcL, editor. *Secretory tumors of the pituitary gland. Progress in endocrine research and therapy,* vol. 1, pp.365-376). New York: Raven Press.

Kramer, A., Saeger, W., Tallen, G. and Ludecke, D. K. (1994). DNA measurement, proliferation markers, and other factors in pituitary adenomas. *Endocr Pathol,* 5, 198-211.

Kubbutat, M. H., Key, G., Duchrow, M., Schluter, C., Flad, H. D. and Gerdes, J. (1994). Epitope analysis of antibodies recognising the cell proliferation associated nuclear antigen previously defined by the antibody Ki-67 (Ki-67 protein). *J Clin Pathol,* 47, 524-528.

Kurki, P., Vanderlaan, M., Dolbeare, F., Gray, J. and Tan, E. M. (1986). Expression of proliferating cell nuclear antigen (PCNA)/cyclin during the cell cycle. *Exp Cell Res,* 166, 209-219.

Landolt, M. A., Shibata, T. and Kleihues, P. (1987). Growth rate of human pituitary tumors. *J Neurosurg,* 67, 803-806.

Lane, D.(1992). P53, guardian of the genome. *Nature,* 358, 15-16.

Levine, A. J., Momand, J. and Finlay, C. A. (1991). The p53 suppressor gene. *Nature,* 315, 453-456.

Lloyd, R.V., Kovacs, K., Young, Jr W.F., Farrel, W.E., Asa, S.L., Truillas, J., Kontogeorgos, G., Sano, T., Scheihauer, B.W., Horvath, E. (2004). Pituitary tumours: Introduction. In: DeLellis RA, Lloyd RV, Heitz PU and Eng C. (Eds.). WHO classification of tumours. Pathology and genetics. Tumours of endocrine organs (pp. 10-13). Lyon, France: IARC Press

Lopez, F., Belloc, F., Dumain, P., Reiffers, J., Bernard, P. and Boisseau, M. R. (1994). The labelling of proliferating cells by Ki-67 and MIB-1 antibodies depends on the binding of a nuclear protein to the DNA. *Exp Cell Res,* 210, 145-153.

Losa, M., Barzaghi, L. A. R , Mortini, P., Franzin, A., Mangili, F., Terreni, M. R. and Giovanelli, M. (2000a). Determination of the proliferation and apoptotic index in adrenocorticotropin-secreting pituitary tumors - Comparison between micro- and macroadenomas. *Am J Pathol,* 156, 245-251.

Losa, M., Franzin, A., Mangili, F., Terreni, M. R., Barzaghi, R., Veglia, F., Mortini, P. and Giovanelli, M. (2000b). Proliferation index of nonfunctioning pituitary adenomas: Correlations with clinical characteristics and long term follow-up. *Neurosurg,* 47, 1313-1319.

Ludecke, D. K., Beck-Bornholdt, H. P., Saeger, W. and Schmidt, W.(1985). Tumor ploidy in DNA histograms of pituitary adenomas. *Acta Neurochir,* 76,18-22.

Maier, H., Morimura, T., Ofner, D., Hallbrucker, C., Kitz, K. and Budka, H. (1990). Argyrophilic nucleolar organizer region proteins (Arg-NORs) in human brain tumors: relations with grade of malignancy and proliferation indices. *Acta Neuropathol* (Berl), 80, 156-162.

Mastronardi, L., Guiducci, A. and Puzzili, F. (2001). Lack of correlation between Ki-67 labelling index and tumor size of anterior pituitary adenomas. *BMC Cancer* 1:12 (http://www.biomedcentral.com/1471-2407/1/12)

Mastronardi, L., Guiducci, A., Spera, C., Puzzili, F., Liberati, F. and Maira, G. (1999). Ki-67 labeling index and invasiveness aming anterior pituitary adenomas: analysis of 103 cases using the MIB-1 monoclonal antibody. *J Clin Pathol,* 52, 107-111.

Mellin, W. (1990). Cytometry in tumor pathology – A critical review of methods and applications, and some results of DNA analysis. *Path. Res. Pract,* 186, 37-62.

Meyer, J. S. and Coplin, M. D. (1988). Thymidine Labeling Index, Flow Cytometric S-Phase Measurement and DNA Index in Human Tumors. *Am J Clin Pathol,* 89, 586-595.

Meyer, J. S., Marchosky, J. A. and Hickey, W. F. (1993). Cell kinetic classification of tumors of the nervous system by DNA precursor labeling in vitro. *Hum Pathol,* 24, 1357-1364.

Mizoue, T., Kawamoto, H., Arita, K., Kurisu, K., Tominaga, A. and Uozomi, T. (1997).
MIB-1 immunopositivity is associated with rapid regrowth of pituitary adenomas. *Acta Neurochir,* 139, 426-432.

Muskhelishvili, L., Latendresse, J. R., Kodell, R. L. and Hederson, E. B.(2003). Evaluation of cell proliferation in rat tissues with BrdU, PCNA, Ki-67 (MIB-5) immunohistochemistry and in situ hybridization for histone mRNA. *J Histochem Cytochem,* 51, 1681-1688.

Nagashima, T., Murovic, J., Hoshino, T., Wilson, C. and DeArmond, S. (1986). The proliferative potential of human pituitary tumors in situ. *J Neurosurg,* 64, 588-593.

Nagashima, T., DeArmond, S. J., Murovic, J. and Hoshino, T. (1985). Immunohistochemical demonstration of S-phase cells by anti-bromodeoxyuridine monoclonal antibody in human brain tumor tissues. *Acta Neuropathol* (Berl), 67, 155-159.

Nakabayashi, H., Sunada, I. and Hara, M. (2001). Immunohistochemical analyses of cell cycle-related proteins, apoptosis and proliferation in pituitary adenomas. *J Histochem Cytochem,* 49, 1193-1194.

Nemoto, R., Uchida, K., Hattori, K., Shimazui, T., Nishijima, Y., Saito, S., Koiso, K. and Harada, M. (1988). S-phase Fraction of Human Bladder Tumor Measured in situ with Bromodeoxyuridine Labeling. *J Urol,* 139, 286-289.

Nishizaki, T., Orita, T., Furutani, Y., Ikeyama, Y., Aoki, H. and Sasaki, K. (1989). Flow-cytometric DNA analysis and immunohistochemical measurement of Ki-67 and BUdR labeling indices in human brain tumors. *J Neurosurg,* 70, 379-384.

Nose-Alberti, V., Mesquita, M. I. S., Martin, L. C. and Kayath, M. J. (1998). Adrenocorticotropin-producing pituitary carcinoma with expression of c-erb-2 and high PCNA index: A comparative study with pituitary adenomas and normal pituitary tissues. *Endocr Pathol,* 9, 53-62.

Pegolo, G., Buckwalter, J. G., Weiss, M. H. and Hinton, D. R. (1995). Pituitary adenomas – Correlation of the cytologic appearance with biologic behavior. *Acta Cytol,* 39, 887-892.

Pernicone, P. J., Scheithauer, B. W., Sebo, T. J., Kovacs, K., Horvarth, E., Young, W. F. Jr, Lloyd, R. V., Davis, D. H., Guthrie, B. L. and Schoene, W. C. (1997). Pituitary carcinoma: a clinicopathologic study of 15 cases. *Cancer,* 79, 804-812.

Pizzaro, C. B., Oliveira, M. C., Coutinho, L. B. and Ferreira, N. P. (2004). Measurement of Ki-67 antigen in 159 pituitary adenomas using the MIB-1 monoclonal antibody. *Braz J Med Biol Res,* 37, 235-243.

Robbins, B. A., De la Vega, D., Ogata, K., Tan, E. M. and Nakamura, R. M. (1987). Immunohistochemical detection of proliferating cell nuclear antigen in solid human malignancies. *Arch Pathol Lab Med,* 111, 841-845.

Saeger, W., Schreiber, S. and Ludecke, D. K. (2001). Cyclins D1 and D3 and topoisomerase II alpha in inactive pituitary adenomas. *Endocr Pathol,* 12, 39-47.

Saeger, W., Ludecke, D. K., Bergmann, M., Schuppert, F., Bosse, U., Herbst, H. and Pagotto, U. (1999). Pituitary carcinoma: definition, incidence, characteristics and case reports. *Pathology, Reseach and Practice,* 195,296. (abstract Nr 78).

Saeger, W. (2004). Proliferation markers and cell inhibitors in pituitary adenomas. *Front Horm Res,* 32, 110-126.

Sambaziotis, D., Kapranos, N. and Kontogeorgos, G. (2003). Correlation of Bcl-2 and Bax with apoptosis in human pituitary adenomas. *Pituitary,* 6, 127-133.

Sanno, N., Teramoto, A., Osamura, Y., Horvath, E., Kovacs, K., Lloyd, V. R. and Scheithauer, B. (2003). Pathology of pituitary tumors. *Neurosurg Clin N Am,* 14, 25-39.

Sasaki, K., Ogino, T. and Takahashi, M. (1986). Immunological determination of labeling index on human tumor tissue sections using monoclonal anti-BrdUrd antibody. *Stain Technology,* 61, 155-161.

Scheithauer, B. W., Kovacs, K. T., Laws, E. R. and Randall, R. V. (1986). Pathology of invasive pituitary tumors with special reference to functional classification. *J Neurosurg,* 65, 733-744.

Schlamp, C. L., Poulsen, G. L., Nork, T. M. and Nickells, R. W. (1997). Nuclear exclusion of wild-type p53 in immortalized human retinoblastoma cells. *J Natl Cancer Inst,* 89, 1530-1536.

Scholzen, T. and Gerdes, J. (2000). The Ki-67 protein : From the known to the unknown. *J Cell Physiol,* 182, 311-322.

Selman, W. R., Laws, E. R. Jr, Scheithauer, B. W. and Carpenter, S. M. (1986). The occurrence of dural invasion in pituitary adenomas. *J Neurosurg,* 64, 402-407.

Shi, S-R., Key, M. E. and Karla, K. L. (1991). Antigen retrieval in formalin-fixed, paraffin-embedded tissues: an enhancement method for immunohistochemical staining based on microwave oven heating of tissue sections. *J Histochem Cytochem,* 39, 741-748.

Shibuya, M., Saito, F., Miwa, T., Davis, R. L., Wilson, C. B. and Hoshino, T. (1992). Histochemical study of pituitary adenomas with Ki-67 and anti-DNA polymerase α monoclonal antibodies, bromodeoxyuridine labeling and nucleolar organizer region counts. *Acta Neuropathol,* 84, 178-183.

Shimon, I. and Melmed, S. (1997). Pituitary tumor pathogenesis. *J Clin Endocrinol Metab,* 82, 1675-1681.

Shivji, K. K., Kenny, M.K. and Wood, R. D. (1992). Proliferating cell nuclear antigen is required for DNA excision repair. *Cell,* 69, 367-374.

Stathopoulou, A., Kaltsas, G., Kontogeorgos, G., Papadogias, D., Makras, P., Kostavaras, K., Gouli, A., Kossivakis, K., Bougiouklis, D., Dimitriou, K., Tsigou, A., Aggelou, A., Seretis, G., and Piaditis, G. (2005). *Expression of Ki-67 antigen in pituitary adenomas:* Correlation with tumor size, invasiveness and function. ECE 2005, Abstract, P2-50, 170-171.

Stefaneanu, L., Murray, D., Kovacs, K. and Smyth, H. S. (1990). Comparative study of DNA content and interphase nucleolar organizer regions in human pituitary adenomas. *Endocr Pathol,* 1, 182-187.

Suhardja, A., Kovacs, K. and Rutka, J. (2001). Genetic basis of pituitary adenoma invasiveness: a review. *J Neurooncol,* 52, 195-204.

Suliman, M., Royds, J., Cullen, D., Timperley, W., Powell, T., Battersby, R. and Jones, T. H. (2001). Mdm2 and the p53 pathway in human pituitary adenomas. *Clin Endocrinol,* 54, 317-325.

Tamatani, R., Taniguchi, Y. and Kawarai, Y. (1995). Ultrastructual study of proliferating cells with an improved immunohistochemical detection of DNA-incorporated bromodeoxyuridine. *J Histochem Cytochem,* 43, 21-29.

Tanaka, Y., Hongo, K., Tada, T., Sakai, K., Kakizawa, Y. and Kobayashi, S. (2003). Growth pattern and rate in residual nonfunctioning pituitary adenomas: correlations among tumor volume doubling time, patient age and MIB-1 index. *J. Neurosurg,* 98, 359-365.

Thapar, K., Yamada, Y., Scheithauer, B., Kovacs, K., Tamada, S. and Stefaneanu, L. (1996a). Assessment of mitotic activity in pituitary adenomas and carcinomas. *Endocr Pathol,* 7, 215-221.

Thapar, K., Scheithauer, B., Kovacs, K., Pernicone, P. and Laws, E. (1996b). p53 Expression in pituitary adenomas and Carcinomas: Correlation with invasiveness and tumor growth fractions. *Neurosurgery,* 38, 765-769.

Thapar, K, Kovacs, K., Scheithauer, B., Stefaneanu, L., Horvath, E., Pernicone, J. P., Murray, D. and Laws, R. E. (1996c). Proliferative activity and invasiveness among pituitary adenomas and carcinomas: an analysis using the MIB-1 antibody. *Neurosurg,* 38, 99-107.

Turner, E. H. and Wass, A. H. J. (1999). Are markers of proliferation valuable in the histological assessment of pituitary tumors? *Pituitary,* 1, 147-151.

Turner, H. E., Nagy, Z. S., Sulliman, N., Esiri, M. M. and Was, J. A. (2000a). Expression analysis of cyclins in pituitary adenomas and the normal pituitary gland. *Clinical Endocrinology,* 53, 337-344.

Turner, H. E., Nagy, Z. S., Gatter, K. C., Esiri, M. M., Wass, J. A. H. and Harris, A. L. (2000b). Proliferation, bcl-2 expression and angiogenesis in pituitary adenomas: relationship to tumor behavior. *Brit J Cancer,* 82, 1441-1445.

Yokoyama, S., Hirano, H., Moroki, K., Goto, M., Imamura, S. and Kuratsu, J. I. (2001). Are nonfunctioning pituitary adenomas extending into cavernous sinus aggressive and/or invasive? *Neurosurgery,* 49, 857-863.

Yonezawa, K., Tamaki, N. and Kokunai, T. (1997). Clinical features and growth fractions of pituitary adenomas. *Surgical Neurology,* 48, 494-500.

Zhao, D., Tomono, Y. and Nose, T. (1999). Expression of p27kip1 and Ki-67 in pituitary adenomas: an investigation of markers of adenoma invasiveness. *Acta Neurochir,* 141, 187-192.

Zuber, P., Hamou, M. F. and De Tribolet, N. (1988). Identification of proliferating cells in human gliomas using the monoclonal antibody Ki-67. *Neurosurg,* 22, 364-368.

In: Focus on Brain Cancer Research
Editor: Andrew V. Yang, pp. 33-46
ISBN 1-59454-973-7

Chapter II

Autocrine or Paracrine Regulation of Pituitary Hormone Production and Secretion by Pituitary Hormone Locally Generated in Human Pituitary Adenomas

Akira Matsuno[1]*, Hideki Katakami[2], Tadashi Nagashima[1], Akira Teramoto[3], R. Yoshiyuki Osamura[4].and Takaaki Kirino[5]

[1] Department of Neurosurgery, Teikyo University Ichihara Hospital, Chiba, Japan
[2] Third Department of Internal Medicine, University of Miyazaki, Faculty of Medicine, Miyazaki, Japan
[3] Department of Neurosurgery, Nippon Medical School, Tokyo, Japan
[4] Department of Pathology, Tokai University School of Medicine, Kanagawa, Japan
[5] Department of Neurosurgery, University of Tokyo Hospital, Tokyo, Japan

Abstract

Historically, there have been two opposing hypotheses concerning the pathogenesis of pituitary adenomas; the hypothalamic hypothesis and the pituitary hypothesis. With the recent demonstration of the monoclonality of most human pituitary adenomas, the pituitary hypothesis, which suggests that pituitary adenomas result from the monoclonal expansion of a single adenohypophyseal cell with subcellular abnormalities, has become the more widely accepted concept. Meanwhile, the role of hypothalamic hormones in the development of pituitary adenomas has recently attracted the attention of investigators

* Correspondence: Akira Matsuno, M.D., Ph.D., Department of Neurosurgery, Teikyo University Ichihara Hospital, 3426-3 Anesaki, Ichihara City, Chiba 299-0111, Japan; Tel: 81-436-62-1211 ext. 2621; Fax: 81-436-62-1357; e-mail: akirakun@med.teikyo-u.ac.jp

once again. In order to confirm the role of locally generated growth hormone-releasing hormone (GHRH) for the progression of somatotroph adenomas, we investigated the expression of GHRH in 25 pituitary somatotroph adenomas immunohistochemically using both conventional avidin-biotin-complex (ABC) method and novel catalyzed signal amplified (CSA) system. In addition, we investigated the expression of GHRH mRNA and GHRH receptor mRNA with in situ hybridization (ISH) using CSA system. The weak immunopositivity of GHRH were observed in only 2 adenomas (8.0%) out of 25 somatotroph adenomas using ABC method. In contrast, 15 adenomas (60.0%) out of 25 somatotroph adenomas were immunopositive for GHRH revealed by CSA system. Very few of non-somatotroph adenomas were immunopositive for GHRH using CSA system. The expression of GHRH mRNA was confirmed using CSA-ISH system in 13 adenomas (72.2%) out of 18 somatotroph adenomas. In 11 adenomas (61.1%) out of 18 somatotroph adenomas, the expression of GHRH receptor mRNA was demonstrated using CSA-ISH system. The demonstration of GHRH and its receptor expression is meaningful in clarifying the autocrine or paracrine regulation of GHRH in GH production and progression of pituitary somatotroph adenomas. Corticotropin-releasing hormone (CRH) expression in corticotroph adenomas, and gonadotropin-releasing hormone (GnRH) expression in human pituitary adenomas were discussed. Such Evidence that indicates endogenous expression of hypothalamic hormones and their receptors in the pituitary and human pituitary adenoma cells has ample significance in autocrine/paracrine regulation of pituitary hormone production.

Key Words: pituitary adenoma, autocrine or paracrine regulation, hypothalamic hormone

Introduction

Historically, there have been two opposing hypotheses concerning the pathogenesis of pituitary adenomas; the hypothalamic hypothesis and the pituitary hypothesis. The hypothalamic hypothesis proposes that pituitary adenomas arise as the downstream consequence of a stimulatory imbalance between hypothalamic hormones emanating from a dysregulated hypothalamus [14, 40, 48, 65]. With the recent demonstration of the monoclonality of most human pituitary adenomas, the pituitary hypothesis, which suggests that pituitary adenomas result from the monoclonal expansion of a single adenohypophyseal cell with subcellular abnormalities such as mutations of coding regions of Gsαprotein [24], has become the more widely accepted concept. Based on this pituitary hypothesis, we have elucidated the cytodifferentiation and cell origins of pituitary adenomas and the functional roles of transcriptional factors working in the cytodifferentiation [32-35, 44, 50-56, 59, 60].

Meanwhile, the role of hypothalamic hormones in the development of pituitary adenomas has recently attracted the attention of investigators once again. For example, growth hormone-releasing hormone (GHRH) production or gene expression in pituitary somatotroph adenomas has been demonstrated by several investigators [20, 26, 36-39, 66, 70]. In recent years, plasma GHRH concentrations in acromegalic patients have been measured in order to investigate the mutual relationship between growth hormone (GH) and GHRH [16, 17, 21, 22]. Among them, we found an extremely rare GHRH-producing pituitary somatotroph adenoma in a 26-year-old acromegalic man with a markedly elevated plasma GHRH concentration [38]. In order to confirm the role of locally generated GHRH for the progression of somatotroph adenomas, we investigated the expression of GHRH in 25 pituitary somatotroph adenomas immunohistochemically and the expression of GHRH mRNA and GHRH receptor mRNA with in situ hybridization (ISH) method. In this chapter, citing the papers of various investigators including ours, we discuss the implications of autocrine or paracrine secretion of three hypothalamic hormones in the development of pituitary adenomas: GHRH expression in somatotroph adenomas [20, 26, 36-39, 66, 70], corticotropin-releasing hormone (CRH) expression in corticotroph adenomas [71], and gonadotropin-releasing hormone (GnRH) expression in human pituitary adenomas [58].

Expression of GHRH, GHRH mRNA, GHRH Receptor mRNA in Pituitary Somatotroph Adenomas

Materials and Methods

We investigated the expression of GHRH, GHRH mRNA and GHRH receptor mRNA histopathologically in 25 somatotroph adenomas from unselected series of 25 acromegalic patients treated in Teikyo University Ichihara Hospital, Chiba, Japan, and University of Tokyo Hospital, Tokyo, Japan. The age distribution of 25 acromegalic patients was from 11 to 72, with mean age of 45.4. Eight male and 17 female patients were included. A basal level of serum GH on admission (normal range: <0.42 ng/ml for men, 0.66-3.68 ng/ml for women) was measured by highly sensitive radioimmunoassay, and the ratios of peak GH and basal GH in thyrotropin-releasing hormone (TRH), GnRH and GHRH provocation tests were calculated. Routinely processed paraffin sections were used for hematoxylin-eosin staining and immunohistochemical staining studies. Paraffin sections were immunostained by an indirect peroxidase method with an antibody against human GH (rabbit, polyclonal, 1:400 diluted in 0.01 M phosphate buffered saline, pH 7.4 (PBS), DAKO, Carpinteria, Ca., U.S.A.), and all the adenomas from 25 acromegalic patients were GH-immunopositive, and they were confirmed to be somatotrophic.

Immunohistochemical Studies of GHRH

Paraffin sections were immunostained with an anti-GHRH antibody corresponding to residues 1-44 amide (rabbit, polyclonal, diluted 1:1000 in 1% bovine serum albumin (BSA)-PBS, UCB Bioproducts, Brussels, Belgium), after the antigen retrieval by microwave irradiation. Immunoreaction was developed both by a conventional avidin-biotin complex (ABC) method using Vectastain's ABC kit (Vector Laboratories Inc., Burlingame, Ca., U.S.A.) and a novel amplified immunohistochemical method using a catalyzed signal amplification (CSA) system (DAKO, Carpinteria, Ca., U.S.A.), and was visualized with diaminobenzidine (DAB) solution containing H2O2. Negative control studies included substituting normal rabbit serum for the primary antibody.

In Situ Hybridization (ISH) Using Catalyzed Signal Amplification (CSA-ISH)

The expression of GHRH mRNA and GHRH receptor mRNA was examined with CSA-ISH using DAKO's GenPoint System (DAKO, Carpinteria, Ca., U.S.A.). The sequence of the biotinylated antisense oligonucleotide probe for GHRH mRNA was 5'-AAG AAC ACC CAG AGT GGC ATC CTT CAC [26], and that of the antisense oligonucleotide probe for GHRH receptor mRNA was 5'-AAA AAG CCC AAA GTT CAC CCC GAC CGA GAG G [57]. The hybridization signals were detected with DAB solution containing H2O2. The negative control experiments carried out were 1) ISH with sense probes, 2) ISH without probes.

Results

Weak immunopositivity of GHRH was observed in only 2 adenomas (8.0%) out of 25 somatotroph adenomas using ABC method. In contrast, 15 adenomas (60.0%) out of 25 somatotroph adenomas were immunopositive for GHRH using CSA system. In order to compare the GHRH immunoreactivity between somatotroph adenomas and the other types of pituitary adenomas, we employed the immunohistochemistry using CSA system for 8 lactotroph, 3 corticotroph, 2 thyrotroph, and 7 endocrinologically inactive adenomas. One out of 8 lactotroph and 1 out of 7 endocrinologically inactive adenomas showed positive immunoreaction for GHRH. None of 3 corticotroph and 2 thyrotroph adenomas was immunopositive for GHRH using CSA system. The details of the immunohistochemical studies were described in our previous reports [36, 37].

The expression of GHRH mRNA was revealed using CSA-ISH system in 13 adenomas (72.2%) out of 18 somatotroph adenomas. In 11 adenomas (61.1%) out of 18 somatotroph adenomas, the expression of GHRH receptor mRNA was confirmed using CSA-ISH system. The details of the in situ hybridization studies were described in our previous reports [36, 37].

We examined the relationship between serum GH, peak/basal GH ratio in GHRH, TRH GnRH provocation tests and GHRH immunopositivity, GHRH mRNA expression. There was no statistically significant difference between serum GH value and GHRH immunopositivity, GHRH mRNA expression. There was no statistically significant difference between peak/basal GH ratios in GHRH, TRH or GnRH provocation test and GHRH immunopositivity, GHRH mRNA expression.

Discussion

Expression of GHRH, GHRH mRNA, GHRH Receptor mRNA in Pituitary Somatotroph Adenomas

GHRH is a well-known hypothalamic hormone that stimulates the synthesis and release of GH as well as the proliferation of GH-producing cells in the anterior pituitary gland [8, 9]. Our present study demonstrated the GHRH production in pituitary somatotroph adenomas, even if GHRH production may be small in amount. GHRH generated by pituitary somatotroph adenomas themselves is considered to be acting as autocrine or paracrine regulator of GH production in the adenomas. GHRH production in somatotroph adenomas implies a possible role of locally generated GHRH in the progression of established somatotroph adenomas. The present study and our identification of a GHRH producing somatotroph adenoma [37] is considered to link the two historically opposing theories, i.e., the hypothalamic hypothesis and the pituitary hypothesis: an established somatotroph adenoma may be developed further by locally produced GHRH through GHRH receptor. Experiments in transgenic mice expressing a human GHRH gene, which suggested existence of the hyperplasia-adenoma sequence, also support linkage of the two theories [43, 67].

Joubert et al. suggested that GHRH synthesis occurred in the normal pituitary and in human GH-producing pituitary adenomas [20]. They measured GH, GHRH, and somatostatin (SRIH) concentrations in the perifusion medium from six somatotroph adenomas and three human pituitaries under basal conditions and in the presence of 10-6 mol/L TRH or SRIH, and their results suggested the release of hypothalamic hormones from pituitary cells. Wakabayashi et al. found GHRH gene expression in six pituitary somatotroph adenomas using the reverse transcription polymerase chain reaction (RT-PCR) [70]. Levy et al. examined 51 human pituitary adenomas for GHRH transcripts using ISH histochemistry, and identified GHRH transcripts in 13 of 17 somatotroph adenomas [26]. Thapar et al. demonstrated accumulation of GHRH mRNA in 91 of a consecutive series of 100 somatotroph adenomas by ISH [66].

Another importance of the overexpression of the GHRH gene in somatotroph adenomas is a prognostically informative event associated with the clinical aggressiveness of somatotroph pituitary tumors. Thapar et al. stated that GHRH transcripts were found to preferentially accumulate among clinically aggressive tumors [66]. In their report, specifically, GHRH mRNA signal intensity was linearly correlated with Ki-67 tumor growth fractions, linearly correlated with preoperative serum GH levels, higher among invasive tumors, and highest in those tumors in which post-operative remission was not achieved. GHRH mRNA signal intensity proved to be the single most significant predictor of postoperative remission. Their data indicate that overexpression of GHRH gene is an event associated with the neoplastic progression and clinical aggressiveness of somatotroph adenomas.

There have been very few reports on GHRH production of non-somatotroph pituitary adenomas in the literature. We examined the GHRH immunoreactivity using CSA system in 8 lactotroph, 3 corticotroph, 2 thyrotroph, and 7 endocrinologically inactive adenomas, and found very few of them, 1 of 8 lactotroph and 1 of 7 endocrinologically inactive adenomas, were immunopositive for GHRH detected with CSA system. None of 3 corticotroph and 2 thyrotroph adenomas was immunopositive for GHRH using CSA system. Levy et al. examined the expression of GHRH mRNA in non-somatotroph pituitary adenomas using ISH histochemistry, and identified GHRH transcripts in 4 of 10 corticotroph, 1 of 6 lactotroph, and 1 of 18 endocrinologically inactive adenomas, whereas GHRH transcripts were identified in 13 of 17 somatotroph adenomas [26]. Both studies found that the positive rates of these non-somatotroph pituitary adenomas were definitely lower than that of somatotroph adenoma. Therefore, GHRH immunopositivity and GHRH mRNA expression are considered to have specific significance for somatotroph adenomas, whereas GHRH production of non-somatotroph pituitary adenomas is still unclear. Lopes et al. demonstrated that GHRH receptor is specifically expressed in somatotroph adenomas, suggesting that GHRH receptor may influence GH release in somatotroph adenomas and may be involved in the growth of somatotroph adenomas [29]. Oka et al. stated that positive signals of GHRH receptor mRNA detected by ISH were observed mainly in somatotroph adenomas and in a few lactotroph adenomas [42]. These results suggest that GHRH receptor plays a role mainly in the function of somatotroph adenomas, and that the function of GHRH receptor in non-somatotroph adenomas such as lactotroph adenomas is still controversial.

GHRH and GHRH receptor production in a somatotroph adenoma has clinical importance in the autocrine or paracrine regulation of GH production and the progression of human somatotroph adenomas through GHRH receptor..

Expression of CRH mRNA in Pituitary Corticotroph Adenomas

The ectopic CRH overproduction of prostate small cell carcinoma, bronchial carcinoid, and gangliocytoma is known to cause the hyperplasia of corticotroph cells [4, 7, 10, 15, 61]. The CRH transgenic mice were found to have high levels of CRH producing corticotroph hyperplasia [64]. Moreover a high level of CRH transcripts has been demonstrated in 17% of 132 pituitary adenomas [27]. Therefore the production of CRH in corticotroph adenoma cells and its implications are to be elucidated. Xu et al. investigated extensively the expression of CRH mRNA in human pituitary corticotroph adenomas [71]. They analyzed 43 corticotroph adenomas from 34 female and 9 male patients: 26 functioning corticotroph adenomas with Cushing's diseases and 17 silent corticotroph adenomas obtained during surgery at the University Hospital of Tokushima, Tokushima, Japan and Toranomon Hospital, Tokyo, Japan, between 1990 and 1998. In their experiments, formalin fixed and paraffin embedded tissues were used for the quantitative CSA-ISH analysis of CRH mRNA with the biotinylated oligonucleotide probe derived from nucleotides 1668-1714 of the human CRH gene (5'-GAG AGC CGC GGG GCT GTC GAG CGA GCG CCG AGG CAG CAG CAG CTG CT-3'). To quantify the CRH mRNA signal intensity in human pituitary corticotroph adenomas, they calculated the percentage of positive CRH mRNA signals within the cytoplasm of tumor cells, and determined the CRH mRNA signal intensity, expressed as the percentage of positive cells of ISH. They also carried out the immunohistochemical stainings of MIB-1 and CRH after the antigen retrieval, using the MIB-1 monoclonal antibody (1:50 dilution;

Immunotech, Marseilles, France) with ABC method and the CRH polyclonal antibody (1:100 dilution; Santa Cruz Biotechnology, Inc., Santa Cruz, Ca., U.S.A.) with CSA method. As a result, they detected, by the CSA-ISH analysis, CRH mRNA signals in 24 of 26 functioning corticotroph adenomas (92.3%), 13 of 17 silent corticotroph adenomas (76.5%) and 6 of 10 normal pituitary glands (60%). They noticed a significant difference in CRH mRNA signal intensity between corticotroph adenomas and normal pituitary glands. They confirmed the cellular localization of CRH protein in corticotroph adenomas with an immunohistochemical method. They also stated that CRH mRNA signal intensity had a significant positive linear correlation with Ki-67 labeling index. Their results can be interpreted that CRH from a local source of corticotroph adenoma cells not only has autocrine/paracrine functions in corticotroph adenomas, but also is an important factor associated with a proliferative potential of human pituitary corticotroph adenomas.

CRH is a hypothalamic hormone that stimulates not only adrenocorticotropic hormone (ACTH) synthesis [12, 68] but also ACTH release by corticotrophs and corticotroph adenoma cells [23, 62]. ACTH secretion and growth of corticotrophs and corticotroph adenoma cells are regulated by other stimulatory agents, such as vasopressin, pituitary leukemia inhibitory factor, and their specific receptors [1, 3, 30, 47], as well as inhibitory factors, such as corticotropin-releasing inhibitory factor and glucocorticoid and its receptor [6, 13, 25]. ACTH secretion is determined by a complex balance of these agents. Xu et al. found no significant linear correlations between higher preoperative plasma ACTH and cortisol levels in the 26 functioning corticotroph adenoma patients and CRH mRNA signal intensity in adenoma cells [71], and stated that the hypercortisolemic state secondary to excess or dysregulated ACTH secretion caused by functioning corticotroph adenoma might not only be determined by CRH from functioning corticotroph adenoma cells themselves, and that plasma ACTH and cortisol levels leading to Cushing's syndrome correlate with a complex balance of several agents.

Expression of GnRH and GnRH Receptor mRNA in Nontumorous and Neoplastic Pituitaries

GnRH is a hypothalamic hormone that stimulates the release and synthesis of luteinizing hormone (LH) and follicle stimulating hormone (FSH) by gonadotroph cells via the GnRH receptor [11, 31]. Recent studies have shown that the presence of GnRH-producing cells [5] and of GnRH mRNA [46] in rat anterior pituitary, which suggests that endogenously synthesized GnRH may be involved in local regulatory mechanisms. Alexander et al. [2] detected GnRH receptor mRNA in human pituitary adenomas in vitro. In addition, using PCR techniques, Miller et al. [41] reported both GnRH and GnRH receptor mRNAs in gonadotroph tumors, as well as in the normal human pituitary. Sanno et al. investigated GnRH and GnRH receptor gene expression in human pituitary adenomas, using recently developed technique of combined ISH and RT-PCR (in situ RT-PCR) methods [58]. In this section, we introduce their studies of the expression of GnRH mRNA and GnRH receptor mRNA in nontumorous human pituitaries and in various types of pituitary adenomas.

They utilized frozen sections of 3 normal autopsy pituitaries, obtained within 8 hr of death from adult patients without endocrine abnormalities, and 33 pituitary adenomas; 5 patients had GH-secreting tumors and acromegaly and elevated serum levels of GH and/or insulin-like growth factor, 4 had prolactin (PRL)-secreting adenomas with elevated serum PRL levels, 3 had ACTH-secreting tumors and Cushing's disease, and 21 had clinically nonfunctioning adenomas with no evidence of hormone hypersecretion and serum PRL levels less than 100 mg/ml. The detailed procedures of the in situ RT-PCR technique, ISH and immunohistochemistry were described in the previous reports [15, 40]. Using RT-PCR, they found GnRH mRNA expressed in normal human pituitaries and in all types of adenomas. Similarly, they noticed GnRH receptor mRNA expressed in nontumorous human pituitaries and in most, but not all, adenomas (5 gonadotroph adenomas, 6 null cell adenomas, 1 of 2 GH-producing tumors, and 1 of 2 ACTH-producing adenomas, but not in the 2 PRL-producing adenomas). Using ISH technique they found GnRH and GnRH receptor mRNAs in all 3 nontumorous pituitaries and in 12 of 33 (36.4%) and 10 of 33 adenomas (30.3%), respectively. Using an indirect in situ RT-PCR technique they detected GnRH and GnRH receptor mRNAs were detected in 29 (87.9%) and 25 (75.8%) of 33 adenomas, respectively. They stated that the presence of GnRH receptor mRNA expression in some GH and ACTH-producing adenomas could explain the abnormal response to GnRH in some patients with acromegaly and Cushing's disease [49, 63]. In their study, GnRH receptor mRNA expression was found in all types of adenomas, except PRL-secreting adenomas, by both RT-PCR and in situ RT-PCR. Although their series include only a small number of tumors of varying type, it is noteworthy that PRL-secreting adenomas did not express GnRH receptor mRNA. Their report is the first report of the localization of GnRH and GnRH receptor mRNAs in individual pituitary adenoma cells using in situ RT-PCR. They concluded that the frequent expression of GnRH and GnRH receptor mRNAs in pituitary cells suggested that GnRH had autocrine/paracrine functions in nontumorous and neoplastic pituitary tissues.

Conclusion

In recent years several investigators have shown the endogenous expression of hypothalamic hormone in the pituitary, as described in this review. A number of other hypothalamic neuropeptides, other than GHRH, CRH and GnRH, that are known to influence anterior pituitary secretion, such as TRH, vasoactive intestinal polypeptide, neuropeptide Y, substance P and galanin have been shown to be synthesized by pituitary cells [18, 19, 28, 45, 69]. The endogenous production of the hypothalamic hormone and its receptor in human pituitary adenoma cells has ample significance in autocrine/paracrine regulation of pituitary hormone production.

References

[1] Akita, S., Webster, J., Ren, S.G., Takino, H., Said, J., Zand, O. and Melmed, S. (1995) Human and murine pituitary expression of leukemia inhibitory factor. Novel

intrapituitary regulation of adrenocorticotropin hormone synthesis and secretion. *J. Clin. Invest* 95;1288-1298.

[2] Alexander, J.M., and Klibanski, A. (1994) Gonadotropin-releasing hormone receptor mRNA expression by human pituitary tumors in vitro. *J. Clin. Invest.* 93:2332-2339.

[3] Antoni, F.A. (1993) Vasopressinergic control of pituitary adrenocorticotropin secretion comes of age. Front. *Neuroendocrinol.* 14;76-122.

[4] Asa, S.L., Kovacs, K., Tindall, G.T., Barrow, D.L., Horvath, E. and Vecsei, P. (1984) Cushing's disease associated with an intrasellar gangliocytoma producing corticotrophin-releasing factor. *Ann. Intern. Med.* 101:789-793.

[5] Bauer, T.W., Moriarty, C.M., and Childs, G.V. (1981) Studies of immunoreactive gonadrotropin releasing hormone (GnRH) in the rat anterior pituitary. *J. Histochem. Cytochem.* 29:1171-1178.

[6] Bilezikjian, L.M. and Vale, W.W. (1983) Glucocorticoids inhibit corticotropin-releasing factor-induced production of adenosine 3',5'-monophosphate in cultured anterior pituitary cells. *Endocrinology* 113;657-662.

[7] Biller, B., Klibanski, A., Koenig, J. and Martin, J.B. (1987) Diagnostic dilemmas in the management of hypothalamic-pituitary-adrenal disorders. *Ann. N. Y. Acad. Sci.* 512:338-350.

[8] Billestrup, N., Swanson, L.W., and Vale, W. (1986) Growth hormone-releasing factor stimulates proliferation of somatotrophs in vitro. *Proc. Natl. Acad. Sci. USA.,* 83: 6854-6857.

[9] Billestrup, N., Mitchell, R.L., Vale, W., and Verma, I.M. (1987) Growth hormone-releasing factor induces c-fos expression in cultured primary pituitary cells. *Mol. Endocrinol.,* 1:300-305.

[10] Carey, R.M., Varma, S.K., Drake, C.R. Jr., Thorner, M.O., Kovacs, K., Rivier, J.and Vale, W. (1984) Ectopic secretion of corticotropin-releasing factor as a cause of Cushing's syndrome. A clinical, morphologic, and biochemical study. *N. Engl. J. Med.* 311:13-20.

[11] Crowley, W.F., Filicori, M., Spratt, D.I., and Santoro, N.F. (1985) The physiology of gonadotropin-releasing hormone (GnRH) secretion in men and women. *Recent. Prog. Horm. Res.,* 41:473-531.

[12] DeBold, C.R., DeCherney, G.S., Jackson, R.V., Sheldon, W.R., Alexander, A.N., Island, D.P., Rivier, J., Vale, W., and Orth, D.N. (1983) Effect of synthetic ovine corticotropin-releasing factor: prolonged duration of action and biphasic response of plasma adrenocorticotropin and cortisol. *J. Clin. Endocrinol. Metab.* 57:294-298.

[13] Engler, D., Redei, E. and Kola, I. (1999) The corticotropin-releasing inhibitory factor hypothesis: a review of the evidence for the existence of inhibitory as well as stimulatory hypophysiotropic regulation of adrenocorticotropin secretion and biosynthesis. *Endocr. Rev.* 20;460-500.

[14] Faglia, G., and Spada, A. (1995) The role of the hypothalamus in pituitary neoplasia. Baillire's. *Clin. Endocrinol. Metab.,* 9:225-242.

[15] Fjellestad-Paulsen ,A., Abrahamsson, P.A., Bjartell, A., Grino, M., Grimelius, L., Hedeland, H. and Falkmer, S. (1988) Carcinoma of the prostate with Cushing's syndrome. A case report with histochemical and chemical demonstration of

immunoreactive corticotropin-releasing hormone in plasma and tumoral tissue. *Acta. Endocrinol* (Copenh). 119:506-516 .

[16] Genka, S., Soeda, H., Takahashi, M., Katakami, H., Sanno, N., Osamura, Y., Fuchinoue, T., and Teramoto, A. (1995) Acromegaly, diabetes insipidus, and visual loss caused by metastatic growth hormone-releasing hormone-producing malignant pancreatic endocrine tumor in the pituitary gland. Case report. *J. Neurosurg.,* 83, 719-723.

[17] Hidaka, H., Hashida, S., Katakami, H., Ishikawa, E., and Matsukura, S. (1992) Sensitive sandwich enzyme immunoassay for human growth hormone-releasing hormone in plasma. *Clin. Chem. Enzym. Comms.,* 4:305-310.

[18] Hsu, D.W., Hooi, S.C., Hedley-Whyte, E.T., Strauss, R.M. and Kaplan, L.M. (1991) Co-expression of galanin and adrenocorticotropic hormone in human pituitary and pituitary adenomas. *Am. J. Pathol.* 138;897-909.

[19] Jones, P.M., Ghatei, M.A., Steel, J., O'Halloran, D., Gon, G., Legon, S., Burrin, J.M., Leonhardt, U., Polak, J.M. and Bloom, S.R. (1989) Evidence or neuropeptide Y synthesis in the rat anterior pituitary and the influence of thyroid hormone status: comparison with vasoactive intestinal peptide, substance P and neurotensin. *Endocrinology* 125;334-341.

[20] Joubert (Bression), D., Benlot, C., Lagoguey, A., Garnier, P., Brandi, A.M., Gautron, J.P., Legrand, J.C. and Peillon, F. (1989) Normal and growth hormone (GH)-secreting adenomatous human pituitaries release somatostatin and GH-releasing hormone. *J. Clin. Endocrinol. Metab.* 68;572-577.

[21] Katakami, H., Hashida, S., Hidaka, H., Ishikawa, E., and Matsukura, S. (1998) Development and clinical application of a highly sensitive enzyme immunoassay (EIA) for human growth hormone-releasing hormone (hGHRH) in plasma. *Endocr. J., 45(Suppl)*:S67-S70.

[22] Kawa, S., Ueno, T., Iijima, A., Midorikawa, T., Fujimori, Y., Tokoo, M., Oguchi, H., Kiyosawa, K., Imai, Y., Kaneko, G., Kuroda, T., Hashizume, K., Osamura, R.Y., and Katakami, H. (1997) Growth hormone-releasing hormone (GRH)-producing pancreatic tumor with no evidence of multiple endocrine neoplasia type 1. *Dig. Dis. Sci.,* 42:1480-1485.

[23] Labrie, F., Gagne, B., and Lefevre, G. (1982) Corticotropin-releasing factor stimulants adenylate cyclase activity in the anterior pituitary gland. *Life. Sci.,* 31:1117-1121.

[24] Landis, C.A., Masters, S.B., Spada, A., Pace, A.M., Bourne, H.R., and Vallar, L. (1989) GTPase inhibiting mutations activate the α chain of Gs and stimulate adenylyl cyclase in human pituitary tumours. *Nature.* 340:692-696.

[25] Leung, D.Y., Hamid, Q., Vottero, A., Szefler, S.J., Surs, W., Minshall, E., Chrousos, G.P. and Klemm, D.J. (1997) Association of glucocorticoid insensitivity with increased expression of glucocorticoid receptor beta. *J. Exp. Med.* 186;1567-1574.

[26] Levy, A. and Lightman, S.L. (1992) Growth hormone-releasing hormone transcripts in human pituitary adenomas. *J. Clin. Endocrinol. Metab.* 74;1474-1476.

[27] Levy, A. and Lightman, S.L. (1993) The pathogenesis of pituitary adenomas. *Clin. Endocrinol* (Oxf). 38;559-570.

[28] Li, J.Y., Knapp, R.J., and Sternberger, L.A. (1984) Immunocytochemistry of a "private" luteinizing-hormone-releasing hormone system in the pituitary. *Cell. Tissue. Res.*, 235:263-266.

[29] Lopes, M.B., Gaylinn, B.D., Thorner, M.O. and Stoler, M.H. (1997) Growth hormone-releasing hormone receptor mRNA in acromegalic pituitary tumors. *Am. J. Pathol.* 150;1885-1891.

[30] Makara, G.B., Kiss, A., Lolait, S.J., and Aguilera, G. (1996) Hypothalamic-pituitary corticotroph function after shunting of magnocellular vasopressin and oxytocin to the hypophyseal portal circulation. *Endocrinology* 137;580-586.

[31] Marshall, J.C., and Kelch, R.P. (1986) Gonadotropin-releasing hormone: role of pulsatile secretion in the regulation of reproduction. *N. Engl. J. Med.,* 315, 1459-1468.

[32] Matsuno, A., Teramoto, A., Takekoshi, S., Utsunomiya, H., Ohsugi, Y., Kishikawa, S., Osamura, R.Y., Kirino, T. and Lloyd, R.V. (1994) Application of biotinylated oligonucleotide probes to the detection of pituitary hormone mRNA using Northern blot analysis, in situ hybridization at light and electron microscopic level. *Histochem. J.* 26;771-777.

[33] Matsuno, A., Teramoto, A., Takekoshi, S., Sanno, N., Osamura, R.Y. and Kirino, T. (1995) Expression of plurihormonal mRNAs in somatotrophic adenomas detected using a nonisotopic in situ hybridization method: Comparison with lactotrophic adenomas. *Hum. Pathol.* 26;272-279.

[34] Matsuno, A., Teramoto, A., Takekoshi, S., Sanno, N., Osamura, R.Y. and Kirino, T. (1995) HGH, PRL and ACTH gene expression in clinically non-functioning adenomas detected with non-isotopic in situ hybridization method. *Endocr. Pathol.* 6;13-20.

[35] Matsuno, A., Sasaki, T., Mochizuki, T., Fujimaki, T., Sanno, N., Osamura, R.Y., Teramoto, A. and Kirino, T. (1996) A case of pituitary somatotroph adenoma with concomitant secretion of growth hormone, prolactin, and adrenocorticotropic hormone: An adenoma derived from primordial stem cell, studied by immunohistochemistry, in situ hybridization and cell culture. *Acta. Neurochir.* 138;1002-1007.

[36] Matsuno, A., Katakami, H., Sanno, N., Ogino, Y., Osamura, R.Y., Matsukura, S., Shimizu, N. and Nagashima, T. (1999) Pituitary somatotroph adenoma producing growth hormone-releasing hormone (GHRH) with an elevated plasma GHRH concentration: A model case for autocrine and paracrine regulation of growth hormone secretion by GHRH. *J. Clin. Endocrinol. Metab.* 84;3241-3247.

[37] Matsuno, A., Katakami, H., Nagashima, T., Teramoto, A., Osamura, R.Y. and Kirino, T. (2000) Growth hormone-releasing hormone (GHRH) expression in pituitary somatotroph adenomas, studied by immunohistochemistry and in situ hybridization using catalyzed signal amplification system. *Hum. Pathol.* 31;789-794.

[38] Matsuno, A., Nagashima, T., Katakami, H., Sanno, N., Teramoto, A., Takekoshi, S., Osamura, R.Y., Kirino, T. and Lloyd, R.V. (2003) Production of pituitary hormone by human pituitary adenoma is under autocrine and paracrine regulation of hypothalamic hormones secreted from adenoma cells. *Acta Histochem. Cytochem.* 36:415-420.

[39] Matsuno, A., Katakami, H., Katayama, H., Nagashima, T., Sanno, N., Teramoto, A., Osamura, R.Y. and Kirino, T. (2003) Autocrine or paracrine regulation of pituitary

hormone secretion by hypothalamic hormone in human pituitary adenomas. *Recent Res. Devel. Human Pathol,* 1:53-62.

[40] Melmed, S. (1992) Etiology of pituitary acromegaly. Endocrinol. *Metab. Clin. North. Am.,* 21:539-551.

[41] Miller, G.M., Alexander, J.M. and Klibanski, A. (1996) Gonadotropin-releasing hormone messenger RNA expression in gonadotroph tumors and normal human pituitary. *J. Clin. Endocrinol. Metab.* 81;80-83.

[42] Oka, H., Kameya, T., Sato, Y., Naritaka, H., and Kawano, N. (1999) Significance of growth hormone-releasing hormone receptor mRNA in non-neoplastic pituitary and pituitary adenomas: a study by RT-PCR and in situ hybridization. *J. Neurooncol.* 41;197-204.

[43] Osamura, R.Y., Oda, K., Utsunomiya, H., Inada, K., Umemura, S., Shibuya, M., Katakami, H., Voss, J.W., Mayo, K.E., and Rosenfeld, M.G. (1993) Immunohistochemical expression of pit-1 protein in pituitary glands of human GRF transgenic mice: its relationship with hormonal expressions. *Endocr. J.,* 40:133-139.

[44] Osamura, R.Y., Tahara, S., Kurotani, R., Sanno, N., Matsuno, A. and Teramoto, A. (2000) Contributions of immunohistochemistry and in situ hybridization to the functional analysis of pituitary adenomas. *J. Histochem. Cytochem.* 48;445-448.

[45] Pagesy, P., Croissandeau, G., Le Dafniet, M., Peillon, F. and Li, J.Y. (1991) Detection of thyrotropin-releasing hormone (TRH) mRNA by the reverse transcription-polymerase chain reaction in the human normal and tumoral anterior pituitary. *Biochem. Biophys. Res. Commun.* 182;182-187.

[46] Pagesy, P., Li, J.Y., Berthet, M. and Peillon, F. (1992) Evidence of gonadotropin-releasing hormone mRNA in the rat anterior pituitary. *Mol. Endocrinol.* 6;523-528.

[47] Ray, D.W., Ren, S.G. and Melmed, S. (1998) Leukemia inhibitory factor regulates proopiomelanocortin transcription. *Ann. N.Y. Acad. Sci.* 840;162-173.

[48] Reichlin, S. (1991) Pathogenesis of pituitary adenomas, In: Faglia G, Beck-Peccoz P, Ambrosi B, Travaglini P, Spada A, Editors. *Pituitary adenomas: New trends in basic and clinical research.* Elsevier Science, Amsterdam, 113-122.

[49] Rubin, A.L. Levin, S.R., Bernstein, R.I., Tyrrell, J.B., Noaco, C., and Forsham, P.H. (1973) Stimulation of growth hormone by luteinizing hormone-releasing hormone in active acromegaly. *J. Clin. Endocrinol. Metab,* 37:160-162.

[50] Sanno, N., Inada, K., Utsunomiya, H., Umemura, S., Itoh, Y., Matsuno, A., Teramoto, A. and Osamura, R.Y. (1994) Expression of Pit-1 product in human pituitaries: histochemical studies using an antibody against synthetic human Pit-1 protein. *Med. Sci. Res.* 22;685-687.

[51] Sanno, N., Teramoto, A., Matsuno, A., Inada, K., Itoh, J. and Osamura, R.Y. (1994) Clinical and immunohistochemical studies on TSH-secreting pituitary adenoma: Its multihormonality and expression of Pit-1. *Modern Pathol.* 7; 893-899.

[52] Sanno, N., Teramoto, A., Matsuno, A., Takekoshi, S. and Osamura, R.Y. (1995) GH and PRL gene expression by nonradioisotopic in situ hybridization in TSH-secreting pituitary adenomas. *J. Clin. Endocrinol. Metab.* 80;2518-2522.

[53] Sanno, N., Matsuno, A., Itoh, J., Kakimoto, K, Teramoto, A. and Osamura, R.Y. (1996) Combined non-isotopic in situ hybridisation and indirect immunohistochemical

analysis of hormone production in the rat pituitary gland. *J. Clin. Pathol.: Mol. Pathol.* 49;M57-M60.

[54] 54. Sanno, N., Teramoto, A., Matsuno, A., Itoh, J., Takekoshi, S. and Osamura, R.Y. (1996) In situ hybridization analysis of Pit-1 mRNA and hormonal production in human pituitary adenomas. *Acta. Neuropathol.* 91;263-268.

[55] Sanno, N., Teramoto, A., Matsuno, A., Takekoshi, S., Itoh, J. and Osamura, R.Y. (1996) Expression of Pit-1 and estrogen receptor messenger RNA in prolactin-producing pituitary adenomas. *Modern Pathol.* 9;526-533.

[56] Sanno, N., Teramoto, A., Matsuno, A. and Osamura, R.Y. (1996) Expression of human Pit-1 product in the human pituitary and pituitary adenomas. *Arch. Pathol. Lab. Med.* 120;73-77.

[57] Sanno, N., Teramoto, A., Osamura, R.Y., Genka, S,. Katakami, H., Jin, L., Lloyd, R.V., and Kovacs, K. 1997. *J. Clin. Endocrinol. Metab,* 82, 2731.

[58] 58.Sanno, N., Jin, L., Qian, X., Osamura, R.Y., Scheithauer, B.W., Kovacs, K., and Lloyd, R.V. (1997) Gonadotropin-releasing hormone and gonadotropin-releasing hormone receptor messenger ribonucleic acids expression in nontumorous and neoplastic pituitaries. *J. Clin. Endocrinol. Metab,* 82:1974-1982.

[59] Sanno, N., Teramoto, A., Sugiyama, M., Matsuno, A., Takumi, I., Tahara, S. and Osamura, R.Y. (1998) Expression of Pit-1 mRNA and activin/inhibin subunits in clinically nonfunctioning pituitary adenomas. *Horm. Res.* 50;11-17.

[60] Sanno, N., Tahara, S., Kurotani, R., Matsuno, A., Teramoto, A. and Osamura, R.Y. (2001) Cytochemical and molecular biological aspects of the pituitary and pituitary adenomas: cell differentiation and transcription factors. *Prog. Histochem. Cytochem.* 36;263-299.

[61] Schteingart, D.E., Lloyd, R.V., Akil, H., Chandler, W.F., Ibarra-Perez, G., Rosen, S.G. and Ogletree, R. (1986) Cushing's syndrome secondary to ectopic corticotropin-releasing hormone-adrenocorticotropin secretion. *J. Clin. Endocrinol. Metab.* 63:770-775..

[62] Sobel, D.O. (1985) Role of cyclic AMP in corticotropin releasing factor mediated ACTH release. *Peptides,* 6:591-595.

[63] Spada, A. and Lania, A. (1996) Hormone receptors in pituitary adenomas. *In Pituitary adenomas,* edited by Landolt, A.M., Vance, M.L. and Reilly, P.L. Churchill Livingstone, pp 59-71.

[64] Stenzel-Poore, M.P., Cameron, V.A., Vaughan, J., Sawchenko, P.E. and Vale, W. (1992) Development of Cushing's syndrome in corticotropin-releasing factor transgenic mice. *Endocrinology* 130;3378-3386.

[65] Thapar, K., Kovacs, K., and Laws, E.R. (1995) The classification and molecular biology of pituitary adenomas. *Adv. Tech. Stand. Neurosurg.,* 22:4-53.

[66] Thapar, K., Kovacs, K.,Stefaneanu, L., Scheithauer, B., Killinger, D.W., Lloyd, R.V., Smyth, H.S., Barr, A., Thorner, M.O., Gaylinn, B. and Laws, E.R.Jr. (1997) Overexpression of the growth-hormone-releasing hormone gene in acromegaly-associated pituitary tumors. An event associated with neoplastic progression and aggressive behavior. *Am. J. Pathol.* 151;769-784.

[67] Umemura, S., Oda, K., Utsunomiya, H., Sanno, N., Itoh, J., Katakami, H. and Osamura, R.Y. (1995) Immunohistochemical characterization of "hyperplasia-adenoma sequence" in the pituitaries of transgenic mice expressing a human growth hormone-releasing factor gene. *Tokai. J. Exp. Clin. Med.* 20;71-79.

[68] Vale, W., Vaughan, J., Smith, M., Yamamoto, G., Rivier, J., and Rivier, C. (1983) Effects of synthetic ovine corticotropin-releasing factor, glucocorticoids, catecholamines, neurohypophysial peptides, and other substances on cultured corticotropic cells. *Endocrinology,* 113:1121-1131.

[69] Vrontakis, M.E., Sano, T., Kovacs, K. and Friesen, H.G. (1990) Presence of galanin-like immunoreactivity in nontumorous corticotrophs and corticotroph adenomas of the human pituitary. *J. Clin. Endocrinol. Metab.* 70;747-751.

[70] Wakabayashi, I., Inokuchi, K., Hasegawa, O., Sugihara, H. and Minami, S. (1992) Expression of growth hormone (GH)-releasing factor gene in GH-producing pituitary adenoma. *J. Clin. Endocrinol. Metab*. 74;357-361.

[71] Xu, B., Sano, T., Yamada, S., Li, C.C. and Hirokawa, M. (2000) Expression of corticotropin-releasing hormone messenger ribonucleic acid in human pituitary corticotroph adenomas associated with proliferative potential. *J. Clin. Endocrinol. Metab.* 85;1220-1225.

In: Focus on Brain Cancer Research
Editor: Andrew V. Yang, pp. 47-68
ISBN 1-59454-973-7

Chapter III

The Extracellular Space of Gliomas: Changes in its Volume, Geometry and Composition during Malignant Progression

Josef Zamecnik,[1*] Lydia Vargova[2,3] and Eva Sykova[2-4]
[1]Department of Pathology and Molecular Medicine, Charles University, 2nd Medical Faculty and University Hospital Motol, Prague, Czech Republic
[2]Dept. of Neuroscience, Charles University, 2nd Medical Faculty, Prague, Czech Republic
[3]Center for Cell Therapy and Tissue Repair, Charles University, 2nd Medical Faculty, Prague, Czech Republic
[4]Institute of Experimental Medicine, Academy of Sciences of the Czech Republic, Prague, Czech Republic

Abstract

The extracellular space (ECS) of the brain is an important microenvironment of nerve cells and a communication channel between neurons and glial cells. Its composition and volume change dynamically during neuronal activity, development, aging, many pathological states such as ischemia, demyelination or trauma and during neoplastic reconstruction of the tissue. It has been suggested that changes in ECS volume and composition also affect the biological behavior of brain tumors. ECS size and geometry can be accurately determined by the tetramethylammonium (TMA^+) real-time iontophoretic method, which uses TMA^+ as an extracellular marker and follows its

[*] Correspondence to: Josef Zamecnik, MD, PhD. Dept. of Pathology and Molecular Medicine, Charles University, 2nd Medical Faculty and University Hospital Motol, V Uvalu 84, 150 06 PRAGUE, Czech Republic; tel: +420 2 2443 5635; fax: +420 2 2443 5620; email: josef.zamecnik@lfmotol.cuni.cz

diffusion in the ECS by the use of ion-selective microelectrodes. In comparison with unaffected brain cortex, experiments have revealed a dramatic increase in the ECS volume of gliomas, correlating with increases in malignancy. However, the diffusion of small molecules in the enlarged ECS of high-grade gliomas is slowed down due to increased macromolecule content. In contrast to low-grade tumors, where the diffusion of molecules is reduced mainly by the presence of a dense network of tumor cell processes, the increase of ECS diffusion barriers in high-grade gliomas is caused by the overproduction of certain components of the extracellular matrix (ECM), mainly of tenascin. These aberrant or "overproduced" ECM glycoproteins not only stabilize the ECS volume, but also serve as a substrate for the adhesion and subsequent migration of tumor cells through the enlarged ECS. Interestingly, these alterations in ECS volume and structure may hinder the diffusion of neuroactive substances and drugs into the neoplastic tissue. The presence of tenascin in the ECS of the neoplasm correlates significantly with increased malignancy and poor clinical outcome of the disease, which makes its immunohistochemical detection useful as a marker for the aggressive biological behavior of tumors.

Introduction

Beside the complex functional changes in tumor cells leading to their proliferation and migration, the expansive and infiltrative growth of glial brain tumors is also enabled by their ability to alter the properties of the surrounding extracellular space (ECS) and to interact with the extracellular matrix. No other human neoplasm carries the morbid implication of a space-occupying lesion as does an expanding and infiltrating glioma because of the limited volume of the cranial vault. Although changes in the geometry of the ECS are thought to be of critical importance for influencing not only the migratory abilities of tumor cells but also the delivery of neuroactive substances and therapeutic drugs into the tumor tissue, there has been only limited information available concerning the structure of the ECS in brain neoplasms. Almost half of the total volume of some gliomas seems to be accounted for by the ECS, and the infiltrative nature of gliomas is wholly dependent upon cell-extracellular matrix (ECM) interactions. Therefore, any current concept of glial neoplasia must incorporate an understanding of the role of the ECS in the biology of gliomas.

Extracellular Space of the Brain Tissue

The ECS of the brain is an important microenvironment of the nervous system, the channel through which nerve cells communicate [54]. The composition of the ECS is complex. The ECS is not filled with a simple salt solution - in the mammalian CNS, the typical ionic constituents of the ECS are basically the same as those of the cerebrospinal fluid, with local changes resulting from neuronal activity [52, 59]. Other important chemical components of the ECS are substances involved in metabolism, particularly glucose and dissolved gases (0_2, and CO_2,). The presence of HCO_3 and CO_2 forms a powerful buffering system that controls extracellular and intracellular pH. The ECS also contains free radical scavengers, such as ascorbate and glutathione, which may counteract some potentially lethal products of oxygen metabolism. In addition, the ECS may contain neurotransmitters - amino acids such as glutamate and aspartate, catecholamines, indolamines such as dopamine and serotonin, various opioid peptides, NO, and growth hormones. Neurotransmitters can be released into the ECS either extrasynapticaly or by escaping from the synaptic cleft ("transmitter spillover"), especially during repetitive stimulation and/or the massive release of neurotransmitter. Transmitter released by spillover can also bind to receptors on nearby synapses, which is described as synaptic crosstalk. The diffusion of neurotransmitters in the ECS and their binding to extrasynaptically located high-affinity binding sites on neurons and glia are the underlying mechanisms of extrasynaptic or "volume" transmission, mediated by diffusion in the extracellular space. This type of communication without synapses provides a way for synchronizing neuronal activity and long-range information processing in functions such as vigilance, sleep, lactation, chronic pain, hunger, depression, long-term potentiation (LTP), long-term depression (LTD), memory formation and other plastic changes in the CNS [58]. The ECS also contains glycosaminoglycans (principally hyaluronate), proteoglycans, and glycoproteins that constitute the extracellular matrix (ECM). These large molecules can slow down the movement (diffusion) of various neuroactive substances through the ECS. More importantly, these molecules can hinder the diffusion of particular neuroactive molecules and ions so that they are confined to certain places, while diffusion in other brain regions will be facilitated.

The structural changes in the CNS occurring under physiological as well as pathological conditions are accompanied by changes in the ECS diffusion parameters. Under physiological conditions, this is particularly evident during nervous tissue development [26, 72] and during aging [55]. Many pathological processes in the CNS are accompanied by a loss of cells or neuronal processes, astrogliosis, demyelination, and changes in the ECM, all of which also critically affect the diffusion of neuroactive substances (for review see [55-57, 63].

Early attempts to use electron microscopy to measure the ECS volume estimated it to be almost non-existent, represented by narrow clefts and small lakes where the ECS widened [6]. However, the diminution in volume seen in these early studies seems to have been an artifact of fixation. Today, electron microscopy methods that preserve the ECS, radiotracer methods and diffusion measurements (see below), all agree that the ECS volume represents on average about 20% of the total brain tissue in the healthy brain (for review see [33]).

Methods to Determine ECS Volume and Structure

To date, several experimental approaches have been developed for analyzing the ECS diffusion parameters. Much of the pioneering work was performed using the radiotracer method, which uses the perfusion of the ECS by radiolabeled compounds that remain in the ECS, such as [^{3}H]inulin, [^{14}C]sucrose or [^{14}C] EDTA [14]; however, the method's practical use is limited by the long perfusion periods, the autolytic processing involved as well as its low applicability for *in vivo* experimental studies. Other methods used to study the ECS *in vivo* have been less comprehensive because they can show only relative changes in ECS volume - these include measurements of tissue resistance [66], integrative optical imaging with the measurement of the apparent diffusion coefficient (ADC) of molecules tagged with fluorescent dye and followed by optical imaging [34], or the analysis of the ADC of water by diffusion-weighted MRI [47, 65]. The most complex and accurate method that allows us to describe and quantify the volume and structure of the ECS in nervous tissue is the real-time iontophoretic method of diffusion analysis.

For many molecules, migration through the ECS is governed by diffusion. The diffusion of "probe" molecules, i.e. molecules that do not cross the cell membrane, can be used to reveal and quantify the structure of the ECS. The diffusion of molecules in the ECS can be described by random motion as they collide with water molecules and occasionally with obstructions such as cell membranes (Figure 1).

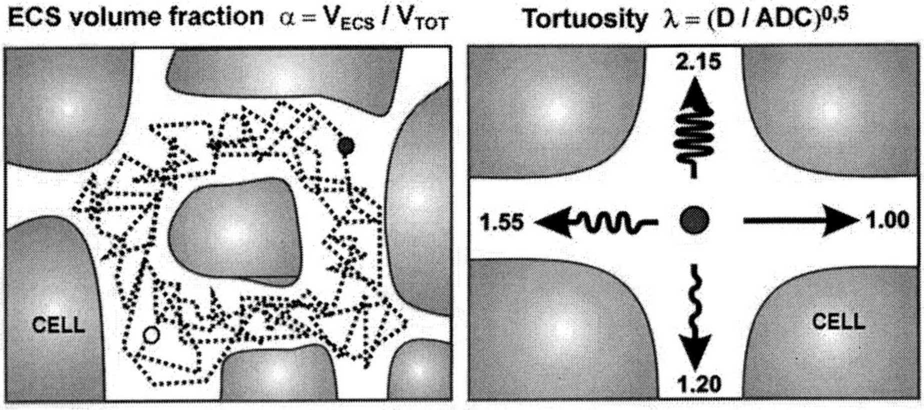

Figure 1. The concept of the extracellular space (ECS) volume fraction (α, *left*) and tortuosity (λ, *right*). V_{ECS}, volume of the ECS; V_{TOT}, total tissue volume; D, free diffusion coefficient; ADC, apparent diffusion coefficient of a substance in tissue. Values of λ correspond to TMA^+ diffusion: 1.00 - free solution, 1.20 - severe brain edema, 1.55 - brain cortex, 2.20 - brain cortex in ischemia. Modified from Sykova [54].

Three ECS diffusion parameters can be obtained from experiments in tumor tissue using the real-time iontophoretic tetramethylammonium (TMA) method:

1. The *extracellular space volume fraction (α)*, which is the ratio between the volume of the ECS and total tissue volume. In comparison with diffusion in a free medium (e.g., in diluted agar), in tissue α is constrained by the restricted volume of the tissue available to diffusing particles; in the healthy brain, α is about 0.2, i.e. the ECS volume fraction is approximately 20% of the total brain volume.
2. The second factor calculated from diffusion measurements is *tortuosity (λ; λ^2=* free/apparent diffusion coefficient), describing the geometric properties of the space available for diffusion, i.e. hindrances slowing down the diffusion of molecules in the ECS. The greater the number of hindrances such as ECM macromolecules or fine neuronal and glial processes, the greater the tortuosity of the ECS, resulting in slower diffusion of an extracellular marker [45, 60]; for review see [11, 55, 56].

3. Nonspecific uptake k′, a factor describing the loss of a substance across cell membranes.

The Real-Time Iontophoretic Method

The absolute values of all three ECS diffusion parameters can be determined by the real-time iontophoretic method developed by Nicholson and Phillips [32]. In brief, an extracellular marker that is restricted to the extracellular compartment is used, such as tetramethylammonium ions (TMA^+, MW = 74.1), to which cell membranes are relatively impermeable. TMA^+ is administered into a tissue slice by iontophoresis, and its concentration in the ECS is measured by a TMA^+-selective microelectrode (Figure 2).

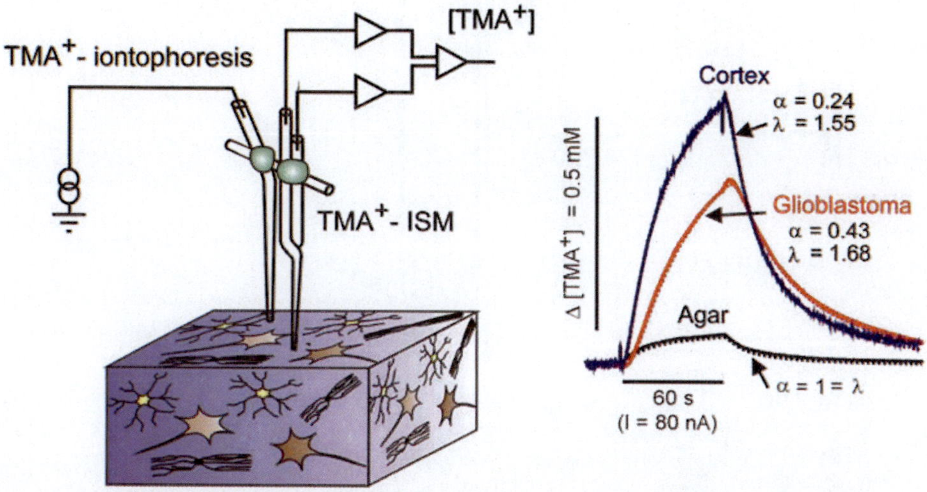

Figure 2. Experimental setup for the measurement of ECS diffusion parameters (*left*) and representative TMA^+-diffusion curves with the corresponding values of the parameters obtained in agar gel, control neocortical tissue and a glioblastoma (*right*). Tetramethylammonium ions (TMA^+) were iontophoresed into the tissue by an iontophoretic micropipette, and their concentration was measured by a TMA^+ ion-selective microelectrode (ISM). Note that the higher the amplitude of the curve, the smaller the value of α; a slower rise and decay indicates a higher tortuosity (λ). In the brain and the tumor, where diffusion is constrained by various barriers and restricted to the extracellular space, the amplitude of the diffusion curve is much higher and its shape differs from the diffusion curve measured in agar gel, where by definition $\alpha = \lambda = 1$ and $k' = 0$. Modified from Zamecnik et al [76]. *α, ECS volume fraction; λ, tortuosity; GB, glioblastoma*

Ion-selective microelectrodes [53] are miniaturized potentiometric sensors that consist of a liquid membrane (liquid ion-exchanger, ion-carrier) placed in the tip (< 3 μm) of a glass micropipette (Figure 3). When introduced into a tissue or calibration solution where ionic activity is to be measured, a Nernst potential develops across the ion-exchanger membrane, i.e., one measures a potential that changes logarithmically with the activity of the ion for which the ion-exchanger is selective. However, when the microelectrode is inserted into neural tissue, it records not only electrical potential differences generated by free ion concentrations, but all types of electrical activity, including membrane, field, action, and synaptic potentials. These confounding factors can be corrected if a reference electrode is in the immediate vicinity of the tip of the ISM. This requirement is best fulfilled by a double-barreled microelectrode, which has a liquid ion-exchanger in one channel while the other channel serves as the reference microelectrode and is, therefore, filled with saline or some other indifferent solution. Because the reference microelectrode also records electrical activity in the tissue, the signal from it is used to cancel out the undesired components.

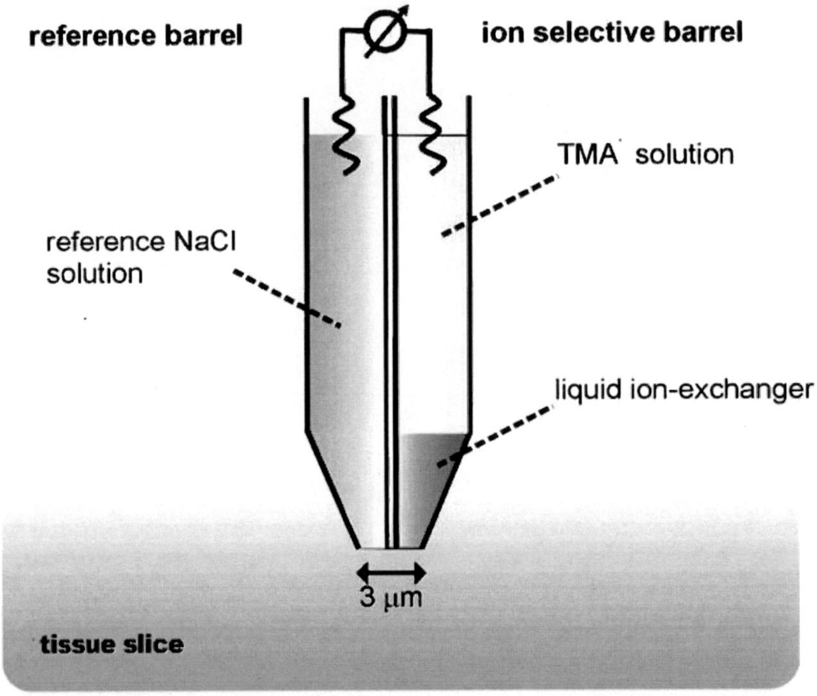

Figure 3. Scheme of a double-barreled TMA^+-selective microelectrode. The tip of the ion-sensitive barrel is filled with a liquid ion exchanger (usually Corning 477317), and the rest of the barrel is back-filled with 100 mM TMA^+ chloride. The reference barrel contains 150 mM NaCl. Adapted from Syková 1992 [53].

For the delivery of TMA^+ into the tissue, an iontophoresis pipette is used, the shank of which is bent before backfilling it with 1 M TMA chloride so that the shank is aligned parallel to that of the ISM. Electrode arrays are made by gluing together an iontophoresis pipette and an ISM with a tip separation of 130 – 200 μm. Typical iontophoresis parameters are +20 nA bias current (continuously applied to maintain a constant transport number), with a +100 nA current step of 40 – 80 s duration to generate the diffusion curve. TMA diffusion curves are captured on a digital oscilloscope and then transferred to a computer, where they are analyzed by fitting the data to a solution of the diffusion equation.

The diffusion parameters (e.g., α, λ and k') can be extracted by a nonlinear curve-fitting simplex algorithm operating on the diffusion curve described by Equation <1> below, which represents the behavior of TMA^+, assuming that it spreads out with spherical symmetry, when the iontophoresis current is applied for duration S. In this expression, C is the concentration of the ion at time t and distance r from the source electrode [32]. The equation governing diffusion in nervous tissue is:

$C = G(t)$ $t < S$, for the rising phase of the curve
$C = G(t) - G(t-S)$ $t > S$, for the falling phase of the curve

The function G(u) is evaluated by substituting t or t-S for u in the following equation:

$$G(u) = (Q\lambda^2 / 8\pi D\alpha r)\,\{\exp[r\lambda(k'/D)^{1/2}]\ \mathrm{erfc}\,[r\lambda/2(Du)^{1/2} + (k'u)^{1/2}] + \exp[-r\lambda(k'/D)^{1/2}]\ \mathrm{erfc}\,[r\lambda/2(Du)^{1/2} - (k'u)^{1/2}]\} \quad (1)$$

The quantity of TMA^+ delivered to the tissue per second is $Q = In/zF$ where I is the step increase in current applied to the iontophoresis electrode, n is the transport number, z is the number of charges associated with the substance iontophoresed (+ 1 here) and F is Faraday's electrochemical equivalent. The function "erfc" is the complementary error function. Knowing n and D, the parameters α, λ and k' can be obtained when the experiment is repeated in a tissue sample. Prior to tissue measurements, diffusion curves are recorded in 0.3% agar gel dissolved in a solution of 150 mM NaCl, 3 mM KCl and 1mM TMA chloride. In dilute agar α and λ are by definition set to 1 and k' is set to 0; the electrode transport number (n) and the free TMA^+ diffusion coefficient (D) are extracted by curve fitting.

It has been repeatedly shown that the *in vitro* ECS diffusion parameters obtained in isolated spinal cords [39] or tissue slices [68] from experimental animals do not differ significantly from those determined *in vivo* [26, 39]. Thus, the data from human tissue slices are assumed to reflect the situation in the human brain *in vivo*, and the results of diffusion experiments provide insight into the dynamic changes in the structure of the space between cells in gliomas.

The Volume of the Extracellular Space in Brain Tumors

Although the characteristic hypercellularity of brain neoplasms would seem to predict a reduced extracellular space in the tumor tissue, a varying degree of ECS enlargement in brain tumors was shown in pioneer electron microscopy studies [2] and in experiments studying the perfusion of radioactively labeled sucrose [3]. Enlarged ECS has been recently confirmed using the TMA^+ iontophoretic method across a spectrum of brain tumors, including astrocytomas, ependymomas, oligodendrogliomas and medulloblastomas [69, 76]. As depicted in Table 1, the extracellular volume fraction α is significantly increased in gliomas (except for oligodendrogliomas), representing almost 48% of the total tissue volume in the most malignant neoplasms. A positive correlation between increasing values of ECS volume fraction and increasing proliferation activity in each distinct histological group of the investigated tumors has also been demonstrated (Figure 4) [69, 76]. Thus, in addition to factors such as the ability of tumor cells to proliferate, adhere and migrate along the existing extracellular matrix [5, 15], the aggressive behavior of tumor cells may also be dependent on the ability of the tumor tissue to create sufficient space for migrating cells.

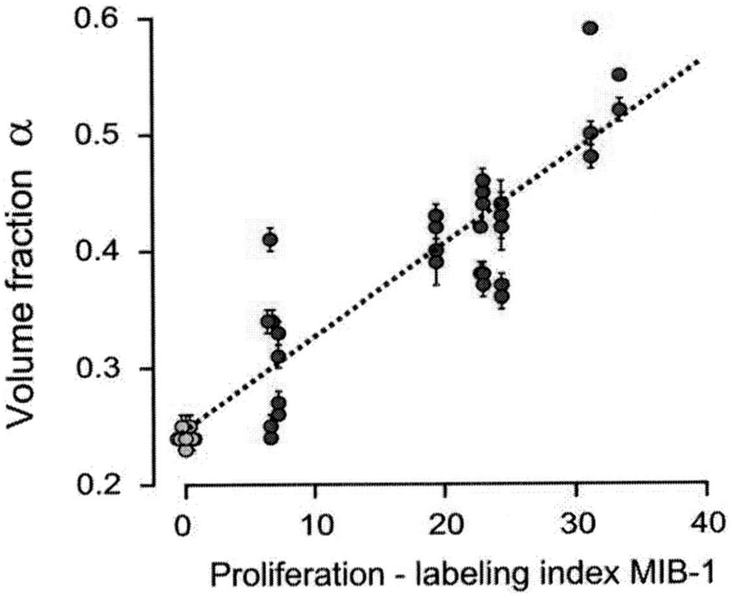

Figure 4. The relationship between the extracellular space volume fraction α and the MIB-1 labeling index (LI) in the studied diffuse astrocytomas (WHO II - IV; *blue circles*). Control data (*yellow circles*) are plotted against MIB-1 LI = 0. Each point represents an average value of α ± S.E.M. calculated from 2 - 3 measurements in different slices. Slices from the same tumor have the same MIB-1 LI values. The regression curve has a correlation coefficient of 0.84. Modified from Vargova et al [69].

Table 1. Results of diffusion measurements in the tissue of brain tumors and in non-affected temporal neocortex

	n	α ± S.E.M.	λ ± S.E.M.
Control temporal neocortex	27	0.24 ± 0.01	1.55 ± 0.03
Pilocytic astrocytomas	36	0.37 ± 0.02*	1.50 ± 0.03
Astrocytomas (grade II)	71	0.29 ± 0.01*	1.57 ± 0.04
Astrocytomas (grade III, IV)	93	0.48 ± 0.01*	1.69 ± 0.03*
Oligodendrogliomas	21	0.23 ± 0.01	1.50 ± 0.02
Ependymomas	22	0.39 ± 0.01*	1.55 ± 0.04
Medulloblastomas - classic	37	0.38 ± 0.03*	1.57 ± 0.04
Medulloblastomas - desmoplastic	20	0.22 ± 0.01	1.85 ± 0.03*

n - number of diffusion measurements; α - ECS volume fraction; λ - ECS tortuosity; S.E.M. - standard error of mean; * significantly increased when compared with control cortex

Therefore, enlargement of the extracellular space accompanies the increased cellularity in non-oligodendroglial gliomas. Several factors may contribute to the enlargement of the ECS. First, the loss of gap junctions between the glioma cells, associated with a decrease in cell-cell communication [51], leads to dysregulation and subsequent decreases in their cellular volume [40]. Secondly, aberrant voltage-dependent as well as ligand-dependent chloride channels in the membranes of glioblastoma cells have been demonstrated [50], which enable a decrease in cellular volume and a shrinkage of the cells through the transport of chloride ions outside the cell, followed by water. The cell volume decrease represents an important factor that enhances the migration of neoplastic cells through the complicated extracellular space. A further decrease in cell volume may also be mediated by complex changes of the surface of the tumor cells and in the length and width of tumor cell processes, as observed in ultrastructural studies [48]. An enlarged ECS volume at the border between a tumor and the surrounding tissue could result from neuronal cell death evoked by the excitotoxic effect of glutamate, which reaches unusually high concentrations in gliomas due to failed glutamate uptake [73]. The ECS volume fraction is not significantly increased in oligodendrogliomas. Glutamine synthetase, the glutamate producing enzyme, is not expressed in oligodendrocytes; hence, these cells may be unable to release excitotoxic glutamate to create more space, as was shown to be the case in astrocytomas [73]. A large extracellular space in high-grade gliomas strongly correlates with the overproduction of extracellular matrix (ECM) macromolecules, especially tenascin and vitronectin [76]. Recent data show that the presence of tenascin is essential for maintaining an optimal distance between cells [61]. The overexpression of large ECM macromolecules in brain tumors, which due to their size and to the mutual repulsion of their highly negatively charged branches occupy a great deal of space and hold cells apart, may therefore significantly contribute to ECS volume enlargement .

Interestingly, the studied pilocytic astrocytomas had, when compared with grade II diffuse astrocytomas, a larger ECS volume fraction in spite of their lower grade and slower growth. This might be due to the enlargement of the ECS by microcysts, which were consistently observed during light microscopic examination of these tumors. The microcysts might be filled by a low-density mucinous fluid without any larger structural glycoproteins, reflecting the low tortuosity of the ECS in these tumors rather than representing an artifact [76].

The Geometry of the Extracellular Space in Gliomas

Diffusion experiments have shown that the increase in the ECS volume in high-grade gliomas is not associated with a decrease in tortuosity but rather with a significant increase in ECS hindrances, which slow the diffusion of small ions [69]. Thus, the newly enlarged ECS in high-grade gliomas does not simply remain empty; the structure of the glioma ECS becomes more complicated than in normal brain tissue. Several factors that could possibly contribute to changes in ECS geometry include cellular density, fibrillary networks of GFAP-

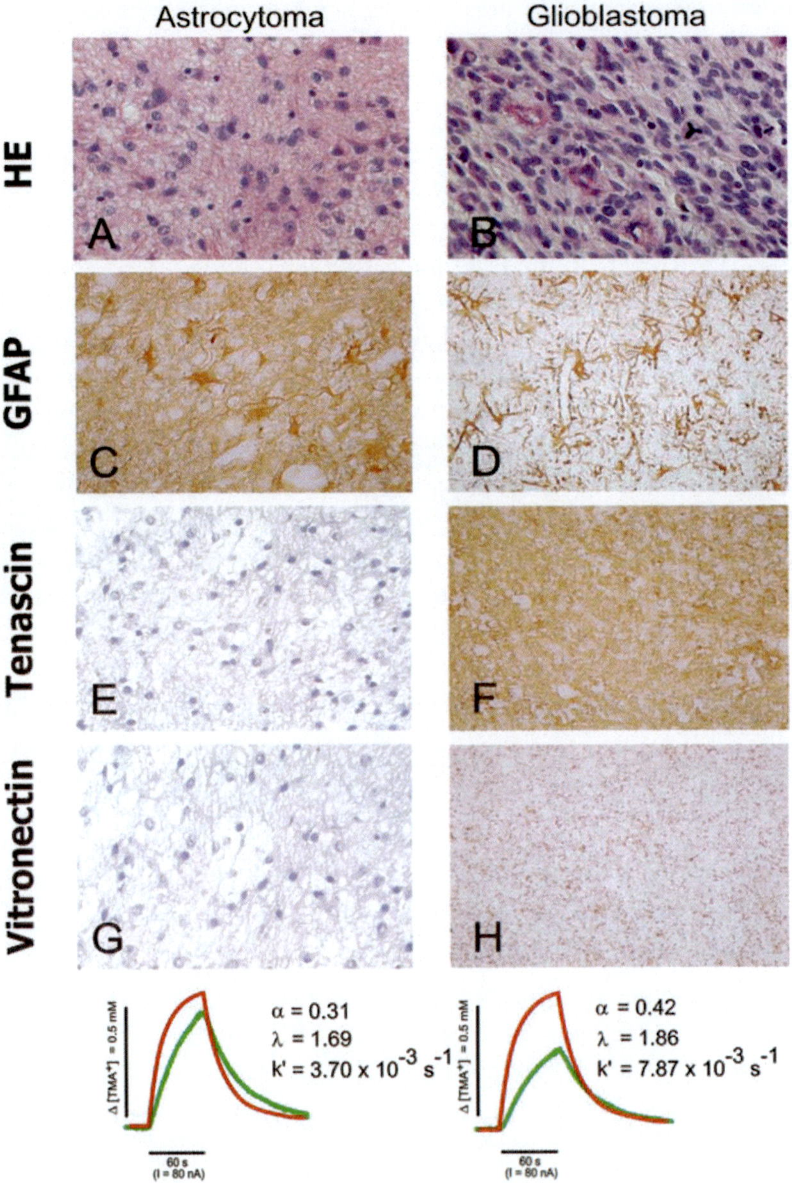

Figure 5. A comparison of tissue structure (A, B; hematoxylin-eosin stain), the density of GFAP-positive tumor cell processes (C, D; immunoperoxidase stain) and the accumulation of tenascin (E, F; immunoperoxidase stain, E counterstained slightly with hematoxylin) and vitronectin (G, H; immunoperoxidase stain, G counterstained slightly with hematoxylin) in the ECS of an astrocytoma (grade II) and glioblastoma (grade IV), along with the ECS diffusion parameters (α, ECS volume fraction; λ, tortuosity). Original magnification 600x.

positive tumor cell processes, hyperplastic tumor vasculature and both qualitative and quantitative changes in the composition of the ECM [76]. Surprisingly, there has been no obvious relation demonstrated between increasing cell density and increasing ECS tortuosity. Furthermore, tortuosity seems to be only slightly influenced by the presence of hyperplastic tumor vasculature. Correlative data indicated that the hindrances to diffusion in the ECS in low-grade gliomas are created by a network of branched processes of the tumor cells. A similar change in ECS tortuosity was also demonstrated in rats as a result of postwounding astrogliosis [45]. In contrast, shortened and less branched tumor cell fibrillary processes are of less importance for ECS tortuosity in high-grade astrocytic tumors, where the major contributor to the tortuosity increase has been shown to be the overproduction of specific ECM glycoproteins [76] (Figure 5).

A paradox arises when considering the increasing number of diffusion barriers in the ECS of the most malignant gliomas, which may also actually potentiate the migratory capacity of the tumor cells. The resolution may lie in the differing requirements of the migration of glioma cells and the movement of small ion. While the movement of both ions and tumor cells is apparently enhanced by an increase in ECS volume, extracellular matrix molecules may simultaneously hinder the diffusion of ions while enhancing cellular movement, since the ECM provides the substrate for tumor cell adhesion and migration.

Diffusion-weighed MRI studies correlating the ADC of water (ADC_w) with tumor grade and the degree of tumor cellularity showed that ADC_w is inversely proportional to the malignancy of the tumor [9, 25, 47]. The authors assumed that a low ADC_w reflects a decrease in ECS volume in hypercellular tumor tissue. However, in experiments using the real-time iontophoretic method, an increase in ECS volume was observed together with an increase in ECS tortuosity and increasing malignancy [69, 76]. In an animal model of nervous tissue injury, it was shown that increased tortuosity due to an increased content of ECM molecules impedes ADC_w without any change in ECS volume [71]. Tortuosity is, by definition, inversely related to ADC; thus, an increase in ECS tortuosity reflects a lower ADC and the slower diffusion of ions and molecules due to diffusion barriers in the tumor environment.

Taken together, the extracellular rearrangement resulting in a net enlargement of the ECS volume along with increased diffusion barriers may prevent the diffusion of regulatory neuroactive and therapeutic substances, resulting in an optimal environment for tumor cell migration, aided and abetted by their capacity to produce metalloproteinases permissive for cellular invasion [41]. Even in the face of increasing intracranial pressure, the most malignant gliomas retain an expanded ECS to the added detriment of the surrounding non-neoplastic brain tissue [76].

Extracellular Matrix in Gliomas

The extracellular matrix is an important component of the microenvironment of the nervous tissue and is involved in both normal and pathological tissue remodeling, such as during development or repair [35]. Moreover, the construction of artificial ECM proteins may be used to control the differentiation of neural stem cells, suggesting a future application for the ECM in neurorestoration and regeneration [28]. Although the ECM of the brain shares most of its components with other human tissues, there are critical differences in its composition: the ECM of the normal brain contains only a limited amount of fibrillary glycoproteins such as collagen or fibronectin, but it contains large amounts of polymerized polysaccharides - glycosaminoglycans and proteoglycans [4, 35].

The presence and potential functions of ECM molecules in brain tumors have been intensively studied (for review see ref. [4]). Although *in vitro* experiments have limitations, the results of experiments in tissue culture give a better understanding of the interactions between tumor cells and the tumoral ECM. The first step in glioma cell migration is thought to be adhesion to ECM components [8]. ECM molecules have also been shown to enhance the mitogenesis of glioma cells [10], being involved in the regulation of cell division leading to a prolongation of their survival [27].

Many ECM glycoproteins such as fibronectin, tenascin, laminin, vitronectin and different types of collagen were shown to be produced by glioma cells in tissue culture and to represent the preferred substrates for the adhesion and migration of glioma cells [4, 16, 18, 37]. However, due to extensive clonal selection and transdifferentiation, mesenchymal features arise in these cultures, with consequent extensive ECM production [30, 38], thus the results obtained by such experiments do not necessarily reflect the situation *in vivo*. Accordingly, substantial differences in ECM composition have been found *in situ* in both astrocytomas [76] and ependymomas [74] in immunohistochemical studies.

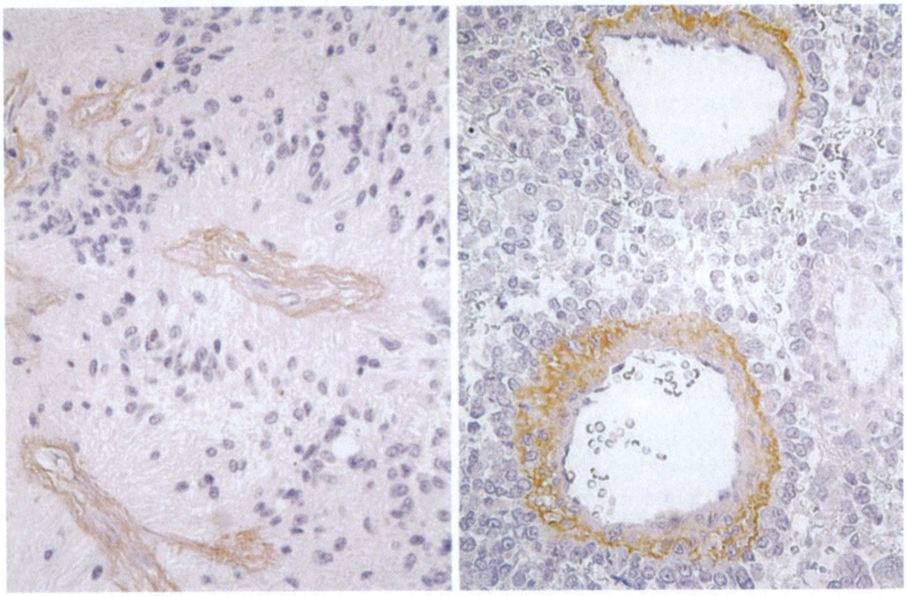

Figure 6. *Left*: Immunoperoxidase staining for laminin localized in the subendothelial basement membranes of hyperplastic blood vessels of a glioblastoma, grade IV (counterstained slightly with hematoxylin). Original magnification 200x. *Right*: Imunoperoxidase staining for type IV collagen in a ependymoma, grade II (counterstained slightly with hematoxylin). Original magnification 200x.

Although the capacity of cultured glioma cells to produce laminin, fibronectin and collagen types I and III-V has been reported [4, 46, 64], no intercellular deposits of these molecules were found by *in situ* studies [74, 76]. In the case of collagen types I and III, their presence was not observed anywhere in the tumor tissue; collagen types IV-VI, laminin and fibronectin were strictly associated with vascular elements of both normal and tumor tissue (Figure 6), independent of the grade of malignancy. Some authors reported a significant decrease in fibronectin [20] or laminin [36] accumulation with increasing tumor grade, but this was not confirmed by others [74, 76]. Moreover, in an experimental model it was shown that the presence of laminin, fibronectin and type IV collagen in gliomas is more likely derived from preexisting blood vessels than from the tumor cells [29]. However, the extensive interstitial production of collagen occurs in rare cases of brain tumors, giving rise to unique entities such as gliofibroma [24], desmoplastic infantile ganglioglioma, desmoplastic cerebral astrocytoma of infancy [67], and desmoplastic glioblastoma [1].

Among ECM glycoproteins, tenascin and vitronectin were detected immunohistochemically in the extracellular matrix surrounding the tumor cells in gliomas. Vitronectin deposits were found in the extracellular matrix of a portion of the most malignant glial tumors [17, 74, 76]. However, the vitronectin production was limited, and a prognostic or diagnostic benefit from its immunodetection could not be demonstrated. In contrast, there was a large amount of tenascin, a large glycoprotein that typically forms a hexabrachion structure [21], detected in both the extracellular matrix and the perivascular tissues of high-grade gliomas (Figure 7). Although tenascin is usually reported as being absent in the developed brain [21], a study of normal brain tissue revealed distinguishable deposits of this glycoprotein in the glial limitans externa, and weak positivity was also detected in the extracellular space of white matter [4, 76]. A correlation between tenascin production and the malignancy or angiogenesis of astrocytomas was clearly demonstrated [19, 23, 36, 42, 76], and the prognostic utility of its immunohistochemical detection has also been extended to ependymomas [74], for which prognostic evaluation by the use of traditional prognostic markers has long been deemed unsatisfactory [75].

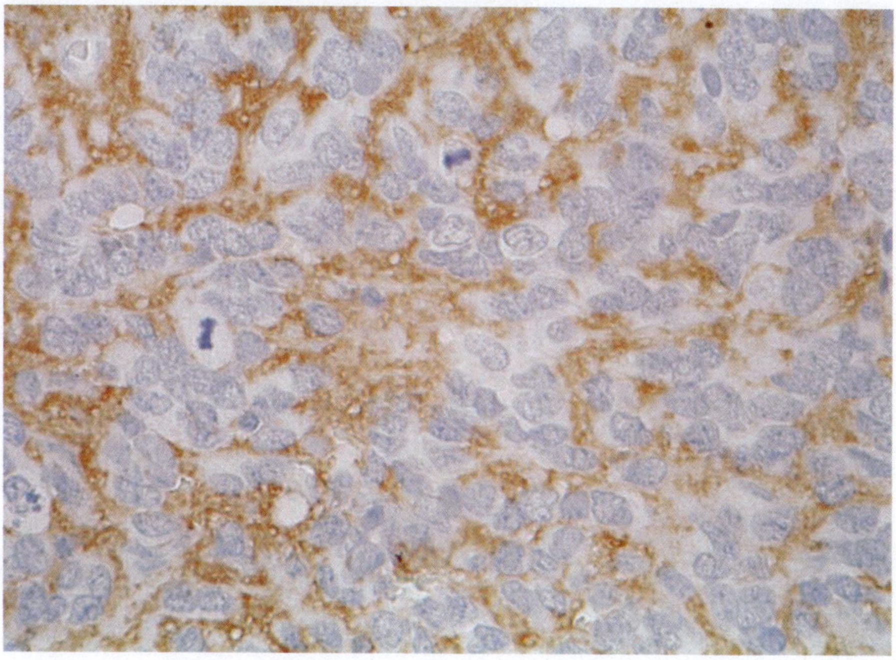

Figure 7. Tenascin-immunopositive deposits in the ECS of a glioblastoma. Immunoperoxidase staining for tenascin (counterstained slightly with hematoxylin, scale bar = 60 μm).

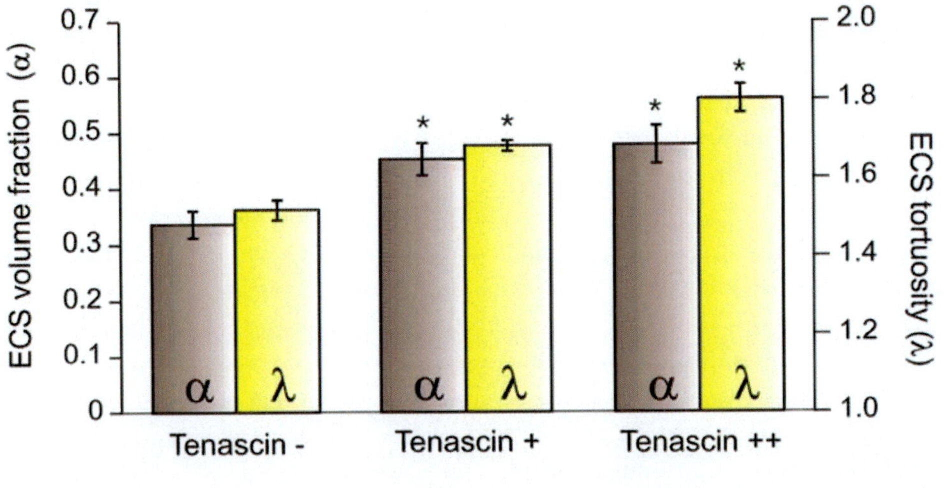

Figure 8. Graphs showing the increase in ECS volume fraction (α) and tortuosity (λ) in astrocytic tumors with a small (tenascin +) or large (tenascin ++) accumulation of tenascin in the ECS, compared to the diffusion parameters of tenascin-negative tumors (tenascin -). Stars indicate significant differences in the diffusion parameters α and λ between tenascin-positive and tenascin-negative tumors. Modified from Zamecnik et al [76].

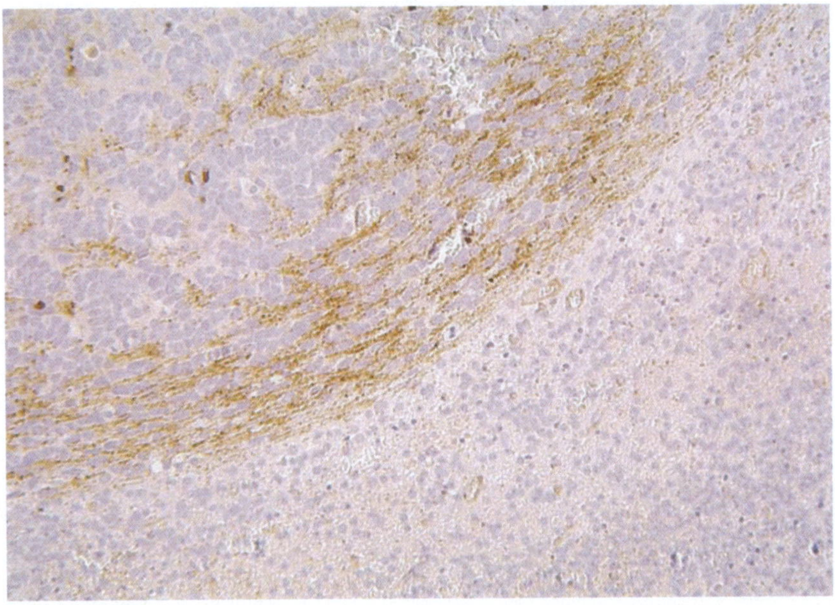

Figure 9. Immunohistochemical demonstration of enhanced tenascin accumulation at the border zones between an ependymoma and the surrounding unaffected tissue. Original magnification 100x.

Based upon correlation with diffusion measurements, the accumulation of tenascin in the ECS of the most malignant glial tumors was suggested to be one of the major factors leading to a critical increase in ECS tortuosity and the simultaneous enlargement of the ECS (Figure 8) [76]. Additional evidence for this hypothesis has come from recent findings of decreased

ECS volume and tortuosity in tenascin knock-out mice [62]. It has also been suggested that the ECM distribution is modified at the brain-tumor zone of confrontation (Figure 9) [29, 74], and the presence of tenascin in the brain-tumor confrontation zone was also shown to represent a negative prognostic factor in pediatric ependymomas [74].

Other components of the brain ECM, such as glycosaminoglycans and proteoglycans, are overexpressed in gliomas, principally hyaluronate, brain enriched hyaluronic acid binding protein (BEHAB/brevican), secreted protein acidic and rich in cystein (SPARC, osteonectin) and many others (for review see ref. [4]). Hyaluronan has been demonstrated to be present in increased amounts in glial tumors [12, 47]. These findings may not necessarily reflect the ability of tumor cells to produce these substances in excess, but rather may reflect the filling of the enlarged ECS by the mucoid ground substances of the brain known to be ubiquitous in the CNS [4]. Also, the ubiquitous presence of hyaluronan in the brain parenchyma does not explain the specific invasion pattern of gliomas along blood vessel walls, white fiber tracts or the subpial glial space.

ECM and Chondroid Metaplasia in Gliomas

The presence of cartilage in neuroepithelial brain tumors has been rarely reported in the literature, and there are many controversies concerning its origin (Figure 10). Kepes et al. [22] observed a smooth transition from glial to chondroid regions in three astrocytomas and one mixed ependymoma-astrocytoma, with a distinct GFAP positivity of both the tumor cells and the chondrocyte-like cells of the cartilage, interpreted as having been derived from the neoplastic astrocytes. Such a transition was not observed in several reported fourth-ventricle ependymomas with inclusions of cartilage nodules [31, 49, 74]. The origin of the cartilage was ascribed in these cases more likely to a metaplastic change of mesenchymal elements, as was once illustrated in the adventitia of a tumor blood vessel [22]. Based upon immunohistochemical analyses of ECM distribution, the mesenchymal cells were believed to share the origin of cartilage with tumor cells capable of synthesizing ECM components. Type II collagen, one of the major structural components of cartilage [13], was demonstrated in a cartilage-containing ependymoma to have accumulated in the wall of tumor blood vessels, in their adventitia as well as in the extracellular matrix of the tumor proper, independent of mesenchymal structures (Figure 11) [74]. In our studies, a similar observation was made for tenascin (Figure 12) and type VI collagen, both of which are also reported to be structural components of human cartilage [7, 70]. The abundant ECM production was accompanied by areas of necroses and dystrophic calcification, in contrast to the other tumors in the series in which the chondroid metaplasia did not develop [74]. Thus, the rare alignment of specific conditions might lead to the formation of chondroid areas, analogous to dystrophic calcification in gliomas. The fact that cartilage areas can occur in glial tumors has a clinical impact - we can avoid considering diagnoses such as teratoma, chondroma or even chondrosarcoma that can be found in the older literature [49].

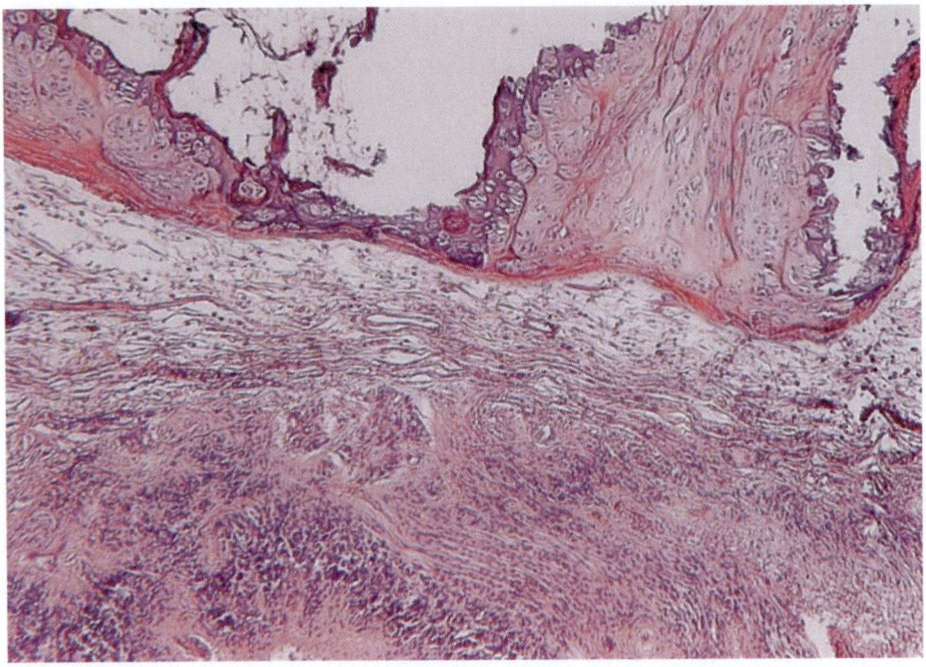

Figure 10. An anaplastic ependymoma of the fourth ventricle containing hyaline cartilage with a formation of metaplastic bone. Hematoxylin-eosin stain; original magnification 2x.

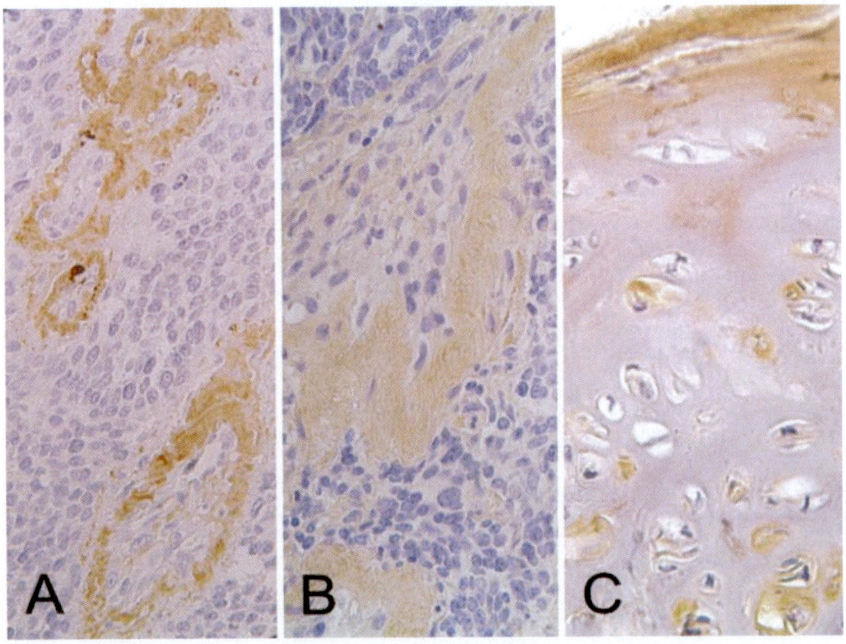

Figure 11. Ependymoma containing a cartilage: immunohistochemical demonstration of type II collagen in the walls of hyperplastic blood vessels (A), in the intersticial collagen bands (B) and in the cartilage (C). Original magnification 400x.

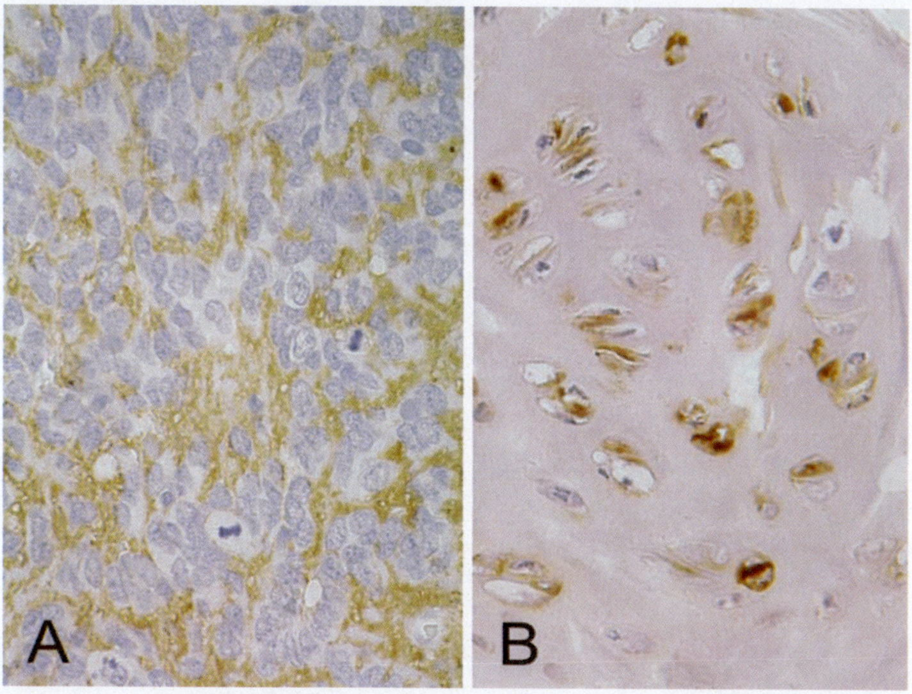

Figure 12. Ependymoma containing a cartilage: immunohistochemical demonstration of tenascin accumulation in both the extracellular space of the tumor (A) and in the cartilage (B). Original magnification 400x.

Conclusion

A growing and relatively recent body of medical literature demonstrates the dynamic changes in both the structure and composition of the extracellular space in brain tumors during their malignant progression. In low-grade gliomas, neoplastic cell processes form a dense network within a slightly enlarged ECS. During the progression to higher grades, the tumor cells gradually loose their capability to regulate their intracellular volume, which then decreases together with a loss of cellular processes; thus, the relative proportion of the ECS in gliomas increases. Cells of the most malignant tumors produce large amounts of tumor-specific ECM components that not only stabilize the ECS volume, but also serve as a substrate for the adhesion and subsequent migration of tumor cells through the enlarged ECS. Additionally, the same changes in structure and composition may hinder the diffusion of neuroactive substances and/or drugs into the neoplastic tissue.

The results concerning the structure of the ECS obtained from diffusion experiments form the basis for future studies. The changes in diffusion parameters and ECM composition may be correlated with the results of *in vivo* examinations by diffusion-weighted MRI and MR spectroscopy, which may in turn lead to enhanced precision in the preoperative grading of gliomas.

Novel therapeutic approaches for the localized delivery of therapeutic agents to brain tumors are being brought to clinical usage [43, 44]. The changes in the volume and composition of the tumor tissue ECS reported in this study, especially in tenascin-positive tumors, are of major importance, as they can critically impair the diffusion of therapeutic agents into tumor tissue and thus may contribute to their reduced effectiveness in some cases. It can be speculated that procedures that would change the ECS structure, i.e. affect the molecules of the ECM, could led to a decrease in ECS volume and reduce the substrate available for cell adhesion and migration. Advances in the understanding of the glioma ECS are critical to therapeutic strategies influencing its structure and composition.

Acknowledgements

The authors wish to thank Prof. Hannes Vogel, M.D., Director of Neuropathology, Stanford University, CA for his critical review of the manuscript.

This project was supported in part by the grant GACR 309/04/0753 from the Ministry of Education of the Czech Republic, the grant VZ FNM 00064203 from the Ministry of Health of the Czech Republic, the grant AV0Z50390512 from the Academy of Sciences of the Czech Republic, and the grant 1M0021620803 from the Ministry of Education of the Czech Republic.

References

[1] Al Sarraj, ST; Bridges, LR. Desmoplastic cerebral glioblastoma of infancy. *Br J Neurosurg,* 1996, 10, 215-219.

[2] Bakay, L. The extracellular space in brain tumours. I. Morphological considerations. *Brain,* 1970, 93, 693-698.

[3] Bakay, L. The extracellular space in brain tumours. II. The sucrose space. *Brain,* 1970, 93, 699-708.

[4] Bellail, AC; Hunter, SB; Brat, DJ; Tan, C; Van Meir, EG. Microregional extracellular matrix heterogeneity in brain modulates glioma cell invasion. *Int J Biochem Cell Biol,* 2004, 36, 1046-1069.

[5] Bolteus, AJ; Berens, ME; Pilkington, GJ. Migration and invasion in brain neoplasms. *Curr Neurol Neurosci Rep,* 2001, 1, 225-232.

[6] Bondareff, W; Pysh, JJ. Distribution of the extracellular space during postnatal maturation of rat cerebral cortex. *Anat Rec,* 1968, 160, 773-780.

[7] Buckwalter, JA; Mankin, HJ. Articular cartilage: tissue design and chondrocyte-matrix interactions. *Instr Course Lect,* 1998, 47, 477-486.

[8] Burg, MA; Nishiyama, A; Stallcup, WB. A central segment of the NG2 proteoglycan is critical for the ability of glioma cells to bind and migrate toward type VI collagen. *Exp Cell Res,* 1997, 235, 254-264.

[9] Castillo, M; Smith, JK; Kwock, L; Wilber, K. Apparent diffusion coefficients in the evaluation of high-grade cerebral gliomas. *AJNR Am J Neuroradiol,* 2001, 22, 60-64.

[10] Chung, CY; Murphy-Ullrich, JE; Erickson, HP. Mitogenesis, cell migration, and loss of focal adhesions induced by tenascin-C interacting with its cell surface receptor, annexin II. *Mol Biol Cell,* 1996, 7, 883-892.

[11] Chvatal, A; Sykova, E. Glial influence on neuronal signaling. *Prog Brain Res,* 2000, 125, 199-216.

[12] Delpech, B; Maingonnat, C; Girard, N; Chauzy, C; Maunoury, R; Olivier, A; Tayot, J; Creissard, P. Hyaluronan and hyaluronectin in the extracellular matrix of human brain tumour stroma. *Eur J Cancer,* 1993, 29, 1012-1017.

[13] Eyre, D. Collagen of articular cartilage. *Arthritis Res,* 2002¨, 4, 30-35.

[14] Fenstermacher, JD; Patlak, CS; Blasberg, RG. Transport of material between brain extracellular fluid, brain cells and blood. *Fed Proc,* 1974, 33, 2070-2074.

[15] Giese, A; Bjerkvig, R; Berens, ME; Westphal, M. Cost of migration: invasion of malignant gliomas and implications for treatment. *J Clin Oncol,* 2003, 21, 1624-1636.

[16] Gladson, CL. The extracellular matrix of gliomas: modulation of cell function. *J Neuropathol Exp Neurol,* 1999, 58, 1029-1040.

[17] Gladson, CL; Cheresh, DA. Glioblastoma expression of vitronectin and the alpha v beta 3 integrin. Adhesion mechanism for transformed glial cells. *J Clin Invest,* 1991, 88, 1924-1932.

[18] Goldbrunner, RH; Bernstein, JJ; Tonn, JC. Cell-extracellular matrix interaction in glioma invasion. *Acta Neurochir* (Wien), 1999, 141, 295-305.

[19] Herold-Mende, C; Mueller, MM; Bonsanto, MM; Schmitt, HP; Kunze, S; Steiner, HH. Clinical impact and functional aspects of tenascin-C expression during glioma progression. *Int J Cancer,* 2002, 98, 362-369.

[20] Higuchi, M; Ohnishi, T; Arita, N; Hiraga, S; Hayakawa, T. Expression of tenascin in human gliomas: its relation to histological malignancy, tumor dedifferentiation and angiogenesis. *Acta Neuropathol* (Berl), 1993, 85, 481-487.

[21] Joester, A; Faissner, A. The structure and function of tenascin in the nervous system. *Matrix Biol,* 2001, 20, 13-22.

[22] Kepes, JJ; Rubinstein, LJ; Chiang, H. The role of astrocytes in the formation of cartilage in gliomas. An immunohistochemical study of four cases. *Am J Pathol,* 1984, 117, 471-483.

[23] Kim, CH; Bak, KH; Kim, YS; Kim, JM; Ko, Y; Oh, SJ; Kim, KM; Hong, EK. Expression of tenascin-C in astrocytic tumors: its relevance to proliferation and angiogenesis. *Surg Neurol,* 2000, 54, 235-240.

[24] Kim, Y; Suh, YL; Sung, C; Hong, SC. Gliofibroma: a case report and review of the literature. *J Korean Med Sci,* 2003, 18, 625-629.

[25] Kono, K; Inoue, Y; Nakayama, K; Shakudo, M; Morino, M; Ohata, K; Wakasa, K; Yamada, R. The role of diffusion-weighted imaging in patients with brain tumors. *AJNR Am J Neuroradiol,* 2001, 22, 1081-1088.

[26] Lehmenkuhler, A; Sykova, E; Svoboda, J; Zilles, K; Nicholson, C. Extracellular space parameters in the rat neocortex and subcortical white matter during postnatal development determined by diffusion analysis. *Neuroscience,* 1993, 55, 339-351.

[27] Liang, Y; Haring, M; Roughley, PJ; Margolis, RK; Margolis, RU. Glypican and biglycan in the nuclei of neurons and glioma cells: presence of functional nuclear

localization signals and dynamic changes in glypican during the cell cycle. *J Cell Biol,* 1997, 139, 851-864.

[28] Liu, CY; Apuzzo, ML; Tirrell, DA. Engineering of the extracellular matrix: working toward neural stem cell programming and neurorestoration--concept and progress report. *Neurosurgery,* 2003, 52, 1154-1165.

[29] Mahesparan, R; Read, TA; Lund-Johansen, M; Skaftnesmo, KO; Bjerkvig, R; Engebraaten, O. Expression of extracellular matrix components in a highly infiltrative in vivo glioma model. *Acta Neuropathol* (Berl), 2003, 105 , 49-57.

[30] Mahesparan, R; Tysnes, BB; Read, TA; Enger, PO; Bjerkvig, R; Lund-Johansen, M. Extracellular matrix-induced cell migration from glioblastoma biopsy specimens in vitro. *Acta Neuropathol* (Berl), 1999, 97, 231-239.

[31] Mathews, T; Moossy, J. Gliomas containing bone and cartilage. *J Neuropathol Exp Neurol,* 1974, 33, 456-471.

[32] Nicholson, C; Phillips, JM. Ion diffusion modified by tortuosity and volume fraction in the extracellular microenvironment of the rat cerebellum. *J Physiol,* 1981, 321, 225-257.

[33] Nicholson, C; Sykova, E. Extracellular space structure revealed by diffusion analysis. *Trends Neurosci,* 1998l, 21, 207-215.

[34] Nicholson, C; Tao, L. Hindered diffusion of high molecular weight compounds in brain extracellular microenvironment measured with integrative optical imaging. *Biophys J,* 1993, 65, 2277-2290.

[35] Novak, U; Kaye, AH. Extracellular matrix and the brain: components and function. *J Clin Neurosci,* 2000, 7, 280-290.

[36] Oz, B; Karayel, FA; Gazio, NL; Ozlen, F; Balci, K. The distribution of extracellular matrix proteins and CD44S expression in human astrocytomas. *Pathol Oncol Res,* 2000, 6, 118-124.

[37] Paulus, W. Brain extracellular matrix, adhesion molecules and glioma invasion. In: Mikkelsen, T; Bjerkvig, R; Laerum, OD; Rosenblum, ML, editors. *Brain Tumor Invasion: Biological, Clinical and Therapeutic Considerations.* New York: Wiley-Liss; 1998; 301-322.

[38] Paulus, W; Huettner, C; Tonn, JC. Collagens, integrins and the mesenchymal drift in glioblastomas: a comparison of biopsy specimens, spheroid and early monolayer cultures. *Int J Cancer,* 1994, 58, 841-846.

[39] Prokopova, S; Vargova, L; Sykova, E. Heterogeneous and anisotropic diffusion in the developing rat spinal cord. *Neuroreport,* 1997, 8, 3527-3532.

[40] Quist, AP; Rhee, SK; Lin, H; Lal, R. Physiological role of gap-junctional hemichannels. Extracellular calcium-dependent isosmotic volume regulation. *J Cell Biol,* 2000, 148, 1063-1074.

[41] Rao, JS. Molecular mechanisms of glioma invasiveness: the role of proteases. *Nat Rev Cancer,* 2003, 3, 489-501.

[42] Rascher, G; Fischmann, A; Kroger, S; Duffner, F; Grote, EH; Wolburg, H. Extracellular matrix and the blood-brain barrier in glioblastoma multiforme: spatial segregation of tenascin and agrin. *Acta Neuropathol* (Berl), 2002, 104, 85-91.

[43] Read, TA; Thorsen, F; Bjerkvig, R. Localised delivery of therapeutic agents to CNS malignancies: old and new approaches. *Curr Pharm Biotechnol,* 2002, 3, 257-273.

[44] Reardon, DA; Akabani, G; Coleman, RE et al. Phase II trial of murine (131)I-labeled antitenascin monoclonal antibody 81C6 administered into surgically created resection cavities of patients with newly diagnosed malignant gliomas. *J Clin Oncol,* 2002, 20, 1389-1397.

[45] Roitbak, T; Sykova, E. Diffusion barriers evoked in the rat cortex by reactive astrogliosis. *Glia,* 1999, 28, 40-48.

[46] Rucklidge, GJ; Dean, V; Robins, SP; Mella, O; Bjerkvig, R. Immunolocalization of extracellular matrix proteins during brain tumor invasion in BD IX rats. *Cancer Res,* 1989, 49, 5419-5423.

[47] Sadeghi, N; Camby, I; Goldman, S et al. Effect of hydrophilic components of the extracellular matrix on quantifiable diffusion-weighted imaging of human gliomas: preliminary results of correlating apparent diffusion coefficient values and hyaluronan expression level. *AJR Am J Roentgenol,* 2003, 181, 235-241.

[48] Scheithauer, BW; Bruner, JM. The ultrastructural spectrum of astrocytic neoplasms. *Ultrastruct Pathol,* 1987, 11, 535-581.

[49] Siqueira, EB; Bucy, PC. Case report. Chondroma arising within a mixed clioma. *J Neuropathol Exp Neurol,* 1966, 25, 667-673.

[50] Sontheimer, H. Malignant gliomas: perverting glutamate and ion homeostasis for selective advantage. *Trends Neurosci,* 2003, 26, 543-549.

[51] Soroceanu, L; Manning, TJ, Jr.; Sontheimer, H. Reduced expression of connexin-43 and functional gap junction coupling in human gliomas. *Glia,* 2001, 33, 107-117.

[52] Sykova, E. Extracellular K+ accumulation in the central nervous system. Prog Biophys *Mol Biol,* 1983, 42, 135-189.

[53] Sykova, E. Ion-selective electrodes. In: Stamford, J, editor. *Monitoring neuronal cells: a practical approach.* New York: Oxford University Press; 1992; 261-282.

[54] Sykova, E. The extracellular space in the CNS: Its regulation, volume and geometry in normal and pathological neuronal function. *Neuroscientist,* 1997, 3, 28-41.

[55] Sykova, E. Glial diffusion barriers during aging and pathological states. *Prog Brain Res,* 2001, 132, 339-363.

[56] Sykova, E. Diffusion properties of the brain in health and disease. *Neurochem Int,* 2004, 45, 453-466.

[57] Sykova, E. Extrasynaptic volume transmission and diffusion parameters of the extracellular space. *Neuroscience,* 2004, 129, 861-876.

[58] Sykova, E. Glia and volume transmission during physiological and pathological states. *J Neural Transm,* 2005, 112, 137-147.

[59] Sykova, E; Chvatal, A. Extracellular ionic and volume changes: the role in glia-neuron interaction. *J Chem Neuroanat,* 1993, 6, 247-260.

[60] Sykova, E; Vargova, L; Prokopova, S; Simonova, Z. Glial swelling and astrogliosis produce diffusion barriers in the rat spinal cord. *Glia,* 1999, 25, 56-70.

[61] Sykova, E; Vorisek, I; Antonova, T et al. Changes in extracellular space size and geometry in APP23 transgenic mice: a model of Alzheimer's disease. *Proc Natl Acad Sci U S A,* 2005, 102, 479-484.

[62] Sykova, E; Vorisek, I; Mazel, T; Antonova, T; Schachner, M. Reduced extracellular space in the brain of tenascin-R and HNK-1 sulfotransferase deficient mice. *Eur J Neurosci,* 2005, in press.

[63] Syková, E; Mazel, T; Vargova, L; Vorisek, I; Prokopova-Kubinova, S. Extracellular space diffusion and pathological states. *Prog Brain Res,* 2000, 125, 155-178.

[64] Tysnes, BB; Mahesparan, R; Thorsen, F; Haugland, HK; Porwol, T; Enger, PO; Lund-Johansen, M; Bjerkvig, R. Laminin expression by glial fibrillary acidic protein positive cells in human gliomas. *Int J Dev Neurosci,* 1999, 17, 531-539.

[65] van der Toorn, A; Sykova, E; Dijkhuizen, RM et al. Dynamic changes in water ADC, energy metabolism, extracellular space volume, and tortuosity in neonatal rat brain during global ischemia. *Magn Reson Med,* 1996, 36, 52-60.

[66] Van Harreveld, A; Dafny, N; Khattab, FI. Effects of calcium on the electrical resistance and the extracellular space of cerebral cortex. *Exp Neurol,* 1971, 31, 358-367.

[67] VandenBerg, SR. Desmoplastic infantile ganglioglioma and desmoplastic cerebral astrocytoma of infancy. *Brain Pathol,* 1993, 3, 275-281.

[68] Vargova, L; Chvatal, A; Anderova, M; Kubinova, S; Ziak, D; Sykova, E. Effect of osmotic stress on potassium accumulation around glial cells and extracellular space volume in rat spinal cord slices. *J Neurosci Res,* 2001, 65, 129-138.

[69] Vargova, L; Homola, A; Zamecnik, J; Tichy, M; Benes, V; Sykova, E. Diffusion parameters of the extracellular space in human gliomas. *Glia,* 2003, 42, 77-88.

[70] Veje, K; Hyllested-Winge, JL; Ostergaard, K. Topographic and zonal distribution of tenascin in human articular cartilage from femoral heads: normal versus mild and severe osteoarthritis. *Osteoarthritis Cartilage,* 2003, 11, 217-227.

[71] Vorisek, I; Hajek, M; Tintera, J; Nicolay, K; Sykova, E. Water ADC, extracellular space volume, and tortuosity in the rat cortex after traumatic injury. *Magn Reson Med,* 2002, 48, 994-1003.

[72] Vorisek, I; Sykova, E. Evolution of anisotropic diffusion in the developing rat corpus callosum. *J Neurophysiol,* 1997, 78, 912-919.

[73] Ye, ZC; Sontheimer, H. Glioma cells release excitotoxic concentrations of glutamate. *Cancer Res,* 1999, 59, 4383-4391.

[74] Zamecnik, J; Chanova, M; Tichy, M; Kodet, R. Distribution of the extracellular matrix glycoproteins in ependymomas - an immunohistochemical study with follow-up analysis. *Neoplasma,* 2004, 51, 214-222.

[75] Zamecnik, J; Snuderl, M; Eckschlager, T; Chanova, M; Tichy, M; Kodet, R. Pediatric intracranial ependymomas: prognostic relevance of histological, immunohistochemical and flow cytometric factors. *Mod Pathol,* 2003, 16, 980-991.

[76] Zamecnik, J; Vargova, L; Homola, A; Kodet, R; Sykova, E. Extracellular matrix and diffusion barriers in human astrocytic tumors. *Neuropathol Appl Neurobiol,* 2004, 30, 338-350.

In: Focus on Brain Cancer Research
Editor: Andrew V. Yang, pp. 69-82
ISBN 1-59454-973-7

Chapter IV

Promising MTH-68/H Oncolytic Newcastle Disease Virus Therapy in Human High Grade Gliomas

Laszlo K. Csatary[1]*, Christine Csatary[1], Georg Gosztonyi[2] and Bela Bodey[3]

[1] United Cancer Research Institute, Alexandria, VA
[2] Institute of Neuropathology, Charité, Universitätsmedizen Berlin, Berlin, Germany
[3] Childrens Center for Cancer and Blood Diseases, Childrens Hospital Los Angeles, and Department of Pathology, Keck School of Medicine, University of Southern California, Los Angeles, CA

Abstract

The employment of virus therapy to treat human neoplasms has a several decade long history. One such virus that has been explored is the Newcastle Disease Virus (NDV), in particular, a therapeutic product named MTH-68/H, derived from an attenuated oncolytic NDV strain. MTH-68/H therapy has been employed in a number of different neoplasms with success. This success has also been demonstrated in glioblastomas and anaplastic astrocytomas. Glioblastoma multiforme (GBM) is the most common primary brain tumor and is by far the most aggressive form of glial tumors. This neoplasm has a poor prognosis, averaging six months to a year. Four cases, presently described, of advanced GBM and anaplastic astrocytoma were treated with the NDV viral product MTH-68/H after the classical modalities of anti-neoplastic therapy had failed. Our results include survival rates of nine and half, to six years, post viral treatment for the surviving patients, and eight years for one patient who has since died, after becoming non-compliant.

* Corresponding author: Laszlo K. Csatáry, M.D. United Cancer Research Institute, 1913 Windsor Road, Alexandria, VA., 22307; Tel: 703 329-7947, Fax: 703 329-0061, E-mail: UCRI@aol.com

Against all odds, these surviving patients returned to a lifestyle that resembles their pre-morbid daily routines. They have been able to enjoy good clinical health. These patients regularly received the MTH-68/H viral therapy for a number of years without interruption as a form of monotherapy once the classical modalities failed. The MRI and CT results have revealed an objective decrease in size of the tumors, in some cases the near total disappearance of the mass. There has also been a documented decrease in mass effect following administration of MTH-68/H. Although one of the four patients described here, did succumb to complications of his malignancy, the results are nonetheless extremely promising in that there is not only a decrease in tumor burden but also a return of pre-morbid functioning. It should be stressed that the positive results may be due to the long-term employment of the oncolytic viral therapy. This chapter seeks to shed light on the background of MTH-68/H with a focus on the possible mechanism of action. There is also a short description of the clinical course of the four cases, as well as of the functional improvement that the patients experienced with the use of MTH-68/H viral therapy after all classical modalities had failed and hope was nearly lost.

Key Words: Glial cell precursors (astrocytes, oligodendrocytes, ependymocytes); Astrocytoma; (ASTR); Glioblastoma (GBM); Neoplasm associated marker (NAM); Neoplasm associated antigen (NAA); Monoclonal antibody (MoAB); Cellular Immunophenotype (CIP); Newcastle Disease Virus (NDV); MTH-68/H, Spontaneous Regression (SR); Monoclonal Antibodies (MoABs), Oncolytic Viral Therapy.

Introduction

"This peculiarity of the membrane, namely, that it becomes continuous with the interstitial matter, the real cement, which binds the nervous elements together and that in all its properties it constitutes a tissue different from the other forms of connective tissue, has induced me to give it a new name, that of neuro-glia (nerve cement)."

Rudolf Virchow, April 3, 1858 [1]

Human Glial Tumors

The most common brain tumors develop from glial cell precursors (astrocytes, oligodendrocytes, ependymocytes). Glial tumors [mainly astrocytomas (ASTRs)], especially glioblastomas, are characterized by hypercellularity, pleomorphism, a number of cell mitoses, cellular immunophenotype (CIP) heterogeneity, various grades of necrosis, and multiple endothelial cell proliferations related to newly generated, tumor-related capillaries. Furthermore, glial tumors are characterized by high grade local invasiveness and a relatively low metastatic tendency. [2-4]

Malignant childhood ASTRs appear within the neuro-glial or macroglial central nervous system (CNS) [5]; they account for over 50% of all intracranial tumors. [3,4,6] Cairncross [7] interpreted the histogenesis of ASTRs in the light of parallel concepts emerging from investigations in myeloproliferative disorders. [8,9] According to the stem cell hypothesis, ASTRs originate from a common pluripotent, neuro-ectodermally derived precursor cell, whose progeny retain the ability to differentiate and do so along astrocytic lines. [10] The majority of malignant glial tumors are incurable with the current classical therapeutical modalities, including surgical resection, radiotherapy, and chemotherapy. [11] This may well be the direct result of the biological variability of these tumors (*e.g.* multiple stem cell lines, intrinsic and acquired multidrug resistance).

The molecular pathogenesis of human brain tumors has been intensely studied during the past few years. Genetic alterations of chromosome 17p are associated with pilocytic ASTRs (World Health Organization (WHO) grade I), mutations at 17p and 19q are common in anaplastic ASTRs (WHO grade III) and abnormal chromosomes 17p, 19q and 10 are associated with the most malignant glioblastoma multiforme (WHO grade IV). [3,12] It is well established that low-grade ASTRs have an intrinsic tendency for progressive immunophenotype (IP) dedifferentiation toward higher-grade, more malignant ASTRs. [13]

Glioblastoma multiforme (GBM), the most malignant neoplasm of the human CNS, develops rapidly *de novo* (primary glioblastoma) or through malignant cellular IP progression from low-grade or anaplastic ASTR (so-called secondary glioblastoma). [14] It was recently reported that mutations of the p53 gene are present in more than two-thirds of secondary glioblastomas, but rarely occur in primary GBMs, suggesting the presence of divergent genetic pathways. [15]

The majority of malignant glial tumors are incurable with the current classical therapeutical modalities. Still the prognosis of high grade gliomas remains somewhat unpredictable because histologic features alone provide an imperfect assessment of the biologic behavior of a given lesion. [16] Whereas some patients experience prolonged disease control after surgery and adjuvant therapy, others with lesions that appear comparable exhibit rapid disease progression and death. Proliferative activity provide a potential correlate of tumorbiologic aggressiveness. [17]

In recent years, there is increasing recognition of polyphenotypic high-grade malignancies in CNS tumor literature. Some of these tumors have been regarded as variants of primitive neuroectodermal tumor (PNET) or as extrarenal malignant rhabdoid tumors (MRTs). Jay and co-workers [18] have described two posterior fossa neoplasms, both of which displayed a "polyphenotypic" expression of neural, epithelial, myogenic, and glial markers. The histological and ultrastructural appearances were inconsistent with glioma, PNET, meningioma, ependymoma, choroid plexus carcinoma, sarcoma, germ cell tumor, and other tumors in the WHO classification. Although the polyphenotype raises the issue that these may represent variants of MRT or the atypical teratoid-rhabdoid tumor, the morphologic findings in the two cases were very dissimilar. The two cases presented by the authors underscore the problems in nosology and classification of polyphenotypic tumors of the CNS. This is particularly significant, as therapeutic protocols for PNET, MRT, and non-CNS polyphenotypic tumors are quite different.

Concurrent viral infections which induce a virus interference phenomenon can significantly modify the outcome of hypothetical viral diseases. [19,20] Participation of one or more viral infections during the intimate steps of the oncogenetic changes was shown in 33% of human cancer. Attenuated (non-pathogenic) avian viruses have been used as a form of non-specific immunobiological, fourth modality treatment of advanced human cancer. The mechanism of viral interference requires the presence of a suitable interfering virus, which is apathogenic to the host and is capable of eliminating the harmful effects of the pathogenic virus. [21,22] We also propose an enhancement of the host tumor-directed immune response induced by the superinfecting apathogenic virus. [23] Detection of *de novo* synthesis of new neoplastic cell associated surface antigens after viral superinfection could also benefit the understanding of this complex immunobiological phenomenon. [24]

Immunosuppression within the Cellular Microenvironment of Childhood Brain Tumors

Important immunological parameter changes have been determined in children suffering from brain tumors: 1) low numbers of circulating T lymphocytes; 2) impaired cytotoxicity of T lymphocyte ($CD8^+$, tumor infiltrating and tumor associated antigen (TAA) directed lymphocytes express a defective high affinity interleukin-2 receptor (IL-2R); 3) poor mitogenic responsiveness of tumor infiltrating T lymphocytes (TIL) *in vitro*; 4) decreased antibody responsiveness (result of defective $CD4^+$ T helper lymphocyte functions); 5) abnormal delayed hypersensitivity responses; and 6) $CD4^+$ and $CD8^+$ lymphocytes derived from TIL are killed by autologous glioma cells *in vitro*. [25,26]

Soluble factors, secreted by brain tumor cells are responsible for the impaired anti-neoplastic cellular immune responses. *In vitro* experiments have revealed that T lymphocytes from normal individuals cultured in the presence of brain tumor cell supernatants exhibit the very same immunological abnormalities mentioned above.

A dominant suppressor growth factor involved in the intratumoral defense mechanisms of neoplastically transformed cells is the transforming growth factor-β2 (TGF-β2). TGF-β2 is derived from primary brain tumors (autocrine secretion), and has been shown to suppress the *in vitro* generation of cytotoxic T lymphocytes (CTL) from TIL derived from peripheral blood lymphocytes [27], and thus its *in vivo* secretion at the tumor site may well be responsible for the intense suppression of $CD8^+$ CTL. [28,29] Brain tumors have been shown to express predominantly low levels of MHC class I molecules, as well as ICAM-1 and to produce TGF-β2, all of which serve as explanations of the inability to effectively isolate and expand infiltrating immunological effectors (CTL) from these neoplasias. This combination of factors probably represents a common tumor biological phenomenon and apparently renders the infiltrating cells incapable of proliferation and considerably lowers their immunological (cytotoxic) efficacy, and may be crucial in the inability of the infiltrating immunological effector cells to overcome tumor progression. [30,31]

Other tumor derived soluble factors, such as prostaglandin E_2 (PGE_2), interleukin-1 receptor (IL-1R) antagonist, and interleukin-10 (IL-10) may also contribute to the observed immunosuppression in childhood brain tumors. [2]

Newcastle Disease Virus (NDV), MTH-68/H

A miracle cannot prove what is impossible,
It is helpful only as confirmation of what is possible.
Maimonides (1135-1204)

The antineoplastic effect of NDV was first published in 1965. [22] In the last three decades, Csatary and co-workers have employed MTH-68/H [19,23,24,32,33,34] an attenuated strain of the Newcastle Disease Virus (NDV), which is harmless to humans. Similar clinically favorable results were also achieved when other attenuated veterinary viruses were employed on several human viral infections. Since the early 1970s, all together 38 viruses have been reported as having had antineoplastic effects on mammalian neoplasms. [21]

Newcastle disease virus (NDV) infects a wide variety of birds and while it can also infect humans, but, in humans it causes only mild flu-like symptoms or conjunctivitis. MTH-68/H contains a unique NDV strain. NDV is classified as an avian paramyxovirus-1 (APMV1), in the *Rubulavirus* genus of the family Paramyxoviridae in the order Mononegavirales. Members of this family have a single stranded, linear, RNA, with an elliptical symmetry. The total genome is roughly 16,000 nucleotides long and contains six genes encoding six major polypeptides: nucleocapsid protein, phosphoprotein, matrix protein, fusion (F) protein, hemagglutinin-neuraminidase (HN), and large RNA-dependent polymerase protein. Replication of the virus takes place in the cytoplasm of the host cell.

Restriction enzyme site mapping of the F protein gene and sequence analysis can be employed to classify the NDV isolates into different genotypes. [35] By this analysis our therapeutic agent, MTH-68/H, contains a strain, which has been proven to belong to a specific genotype group. Studies have demonstrated the remarkable genetic stability of the viral strain contained in MTH-68/H, even after prolonged passage. [36]

The perception that some NDV strains can replicate up to 10,000 times better in human neoplastically transformed cells than in most normal human cells (and the widely accepted fact that the virus is non-toxic) aroused the interest in its use as a form of cancer therapy.

The NDV strains believed to be suitable for antineoplastic therapy can be further classified as either lytic or nonlytic for human cells. Lytic strains and nonlytic strains both appear to replicate much more efficiently in human neoplastic cells than they do in most normal human cells and viruses of both strain types have been investigated as potential anticancer agents. One major difference between lytic strains and nonlytic strains is that lytic strains are able to make infectious progeny virus particles in human cells, whereas nonlytic strains are not. The progeny virus particles made by nonlytic strains contain inactive versions of these molecules. The production of infectious progeny virus particles by lytic strains gives them the ability to kill host cells fairly quickly.

In NDV therapeutics, the strains that have been evaluated most widely for the treatment of human neoplasms are those represented by MTH-68/H, PV-701, 73-T and Ulster. The first three are lytic while Ulster is nonlytic.

Among the few real potentially effective NDV strains evaluated for the treatment of cancer MTH-68/H is unique. MTH-68/H, the medicinal product, contains a highly purified attenuated live NDV virus strain which has been developed to be suitable for intravenous patient administration. The product is freeze dried with specific innocuous stabilizers assuring the long-term stability of the finished product.

The other specificity of MTH-68/H, as an oncolytic strain, is that these viruses can destroy their host cells: (1) by inducing *necrosis* or *lysis* by their excessive replication; (2) by inducing programmed cell death, *apoptosis*. [37] The replication competent MTH-68/H virus therapeutic agent selectively targets neoplastically transformed cells and destroys their host tumour cells while leaving the normal cells uninfected. [37,38] The MTH-68/H strain's safety is extensively proven as well as the excellent tolerability by patients with minimal, if any, side effects.

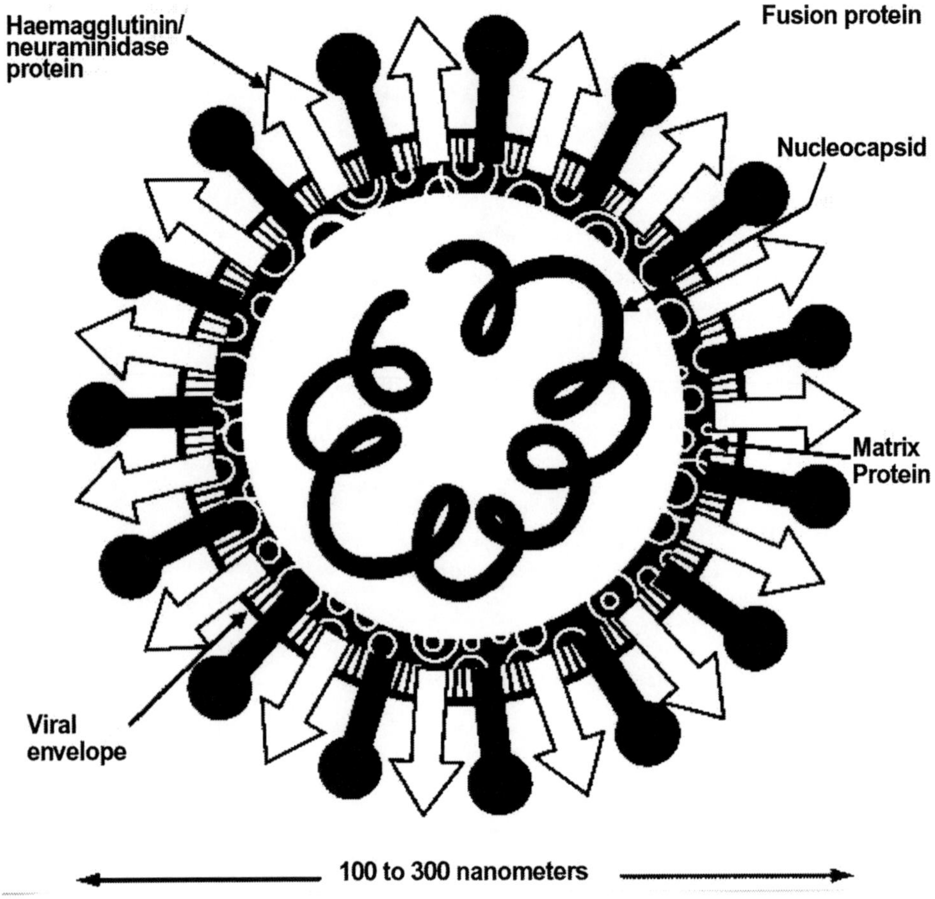

Significant changes appear in the clinical laboratory parameters (tumor markers, liver transaminases and other enzymes, blood cells) following the treatment with NDV derived MTH-68/H, demonstrating a stop or slow down in the progression of the primary cancer disease. A significant number of the cases of primary and metastatic tumors had a partial or total regression after MTH-68/H was employed. [32] Some patients classified in the stage of advanced neoplastic disease were later determined to be in a tumor free clinical condition.

Case Studies

Below, we provide a short description of four cases of high grade gliomas treated with MTH-68/H.

Case 1

This is a 23-year-old male with a left fronto-temporal GBM. Conventional therapy could not prevent recurrence. MTH-68/H therapy resulted in continuous regression of his tumor. In 2002 only residual changes could be shown. Since 1998 the patient drives a car, has graduated from college, and now attends university.

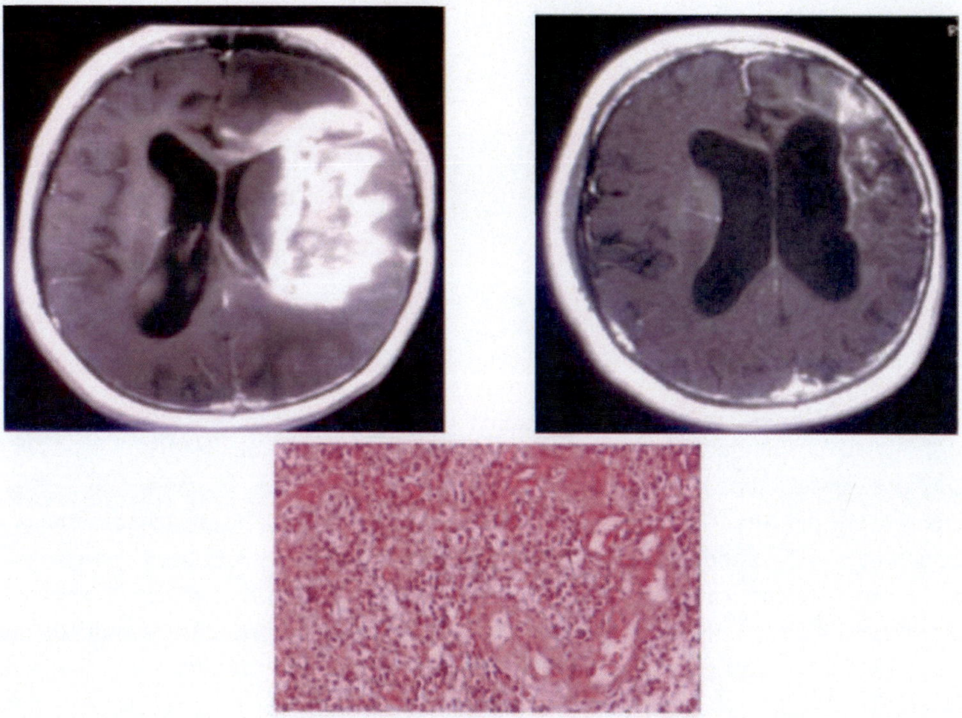

Case 1

Case 2

This is a 22-year-old female, operated on because of a left fronto-temporal glioma, WHO Grade III/IV. Severe progression occurred despite radio- and chemotherapy and reoperation. Institution of MTH-68/H therapy was followed by a dramatic improvement, with almost complete disappearance of the tumor. In 2000, only residual changes could be displayed. She presently attends college.

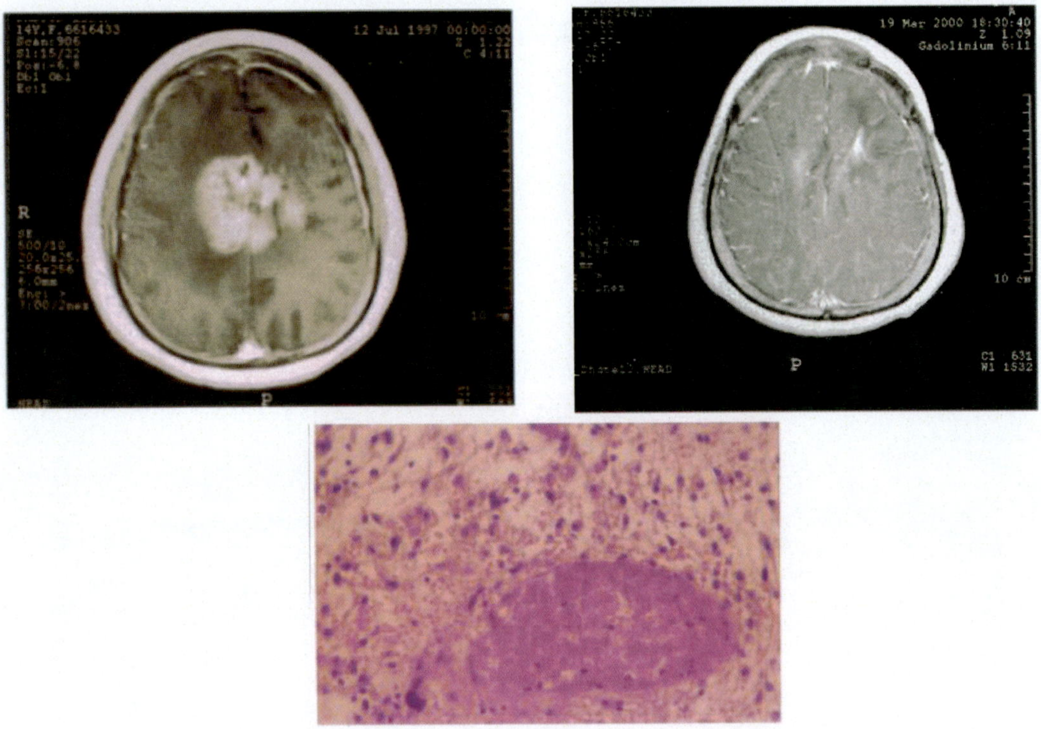

Case 2

Case 3

This case is that of a boy. In 1996, a left temporo-parietal GBM was partially resected. In spite of intense chemotherapy, there was severe tumor progression. In 1997 i.v. MTH-68/H therapy was started, leading to significant clinical improvement. In 1998 two stereotactic resections were performed because of focal recurrences. Despite these reoccurrences since 2002 a stable clinical condition with ongoing MTH-68/H therapy had been achieved for six years, using solely surgical interventions, and viral therapy. While his case did not achieve full remission with viral therapy, his clinical condition dramatically improved, and he remained stable. The patient however, unfortunately became non compliant in 2004, and died in May 2005 .

Case 4

This case is that of a 49-year-old woman. In 1998, there was a partial resection of a bi-frontal GBM, followed by intense chemotherapy and radiation. MTH-68-H therapy was started as sole therapy in 1999. From 2000, there was gradual improvement concomitant with reduction of the tumor mass. For five years, after beginning viral therapy the patient remained stable and was able to partake in daily activities. In 2005 the patient had tumor reoccurrence, and has subsequently stopped any form of therapy.

1998

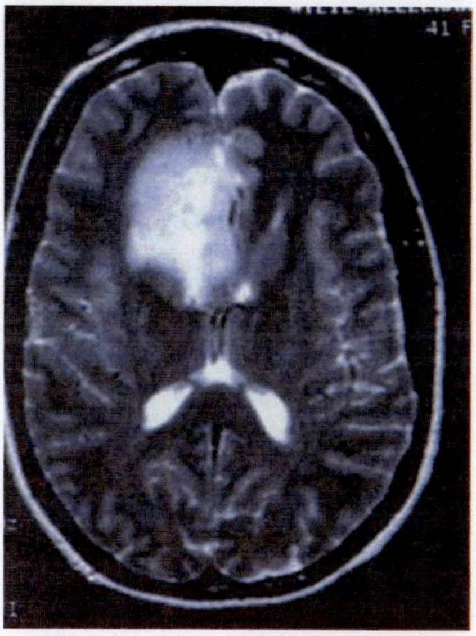

2000

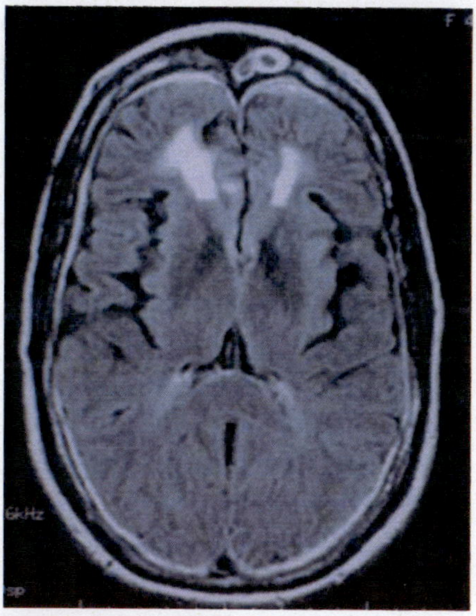

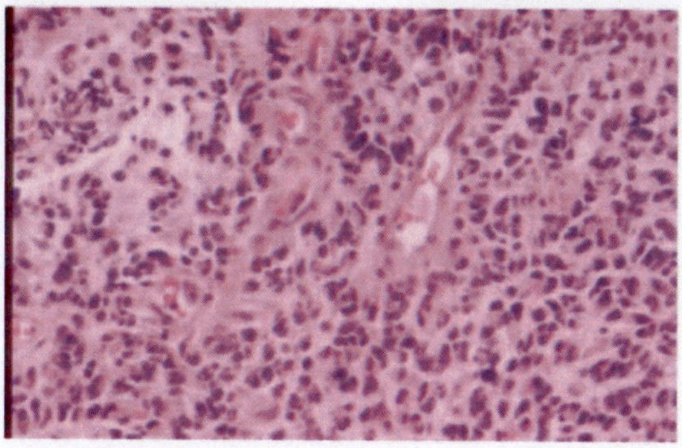

Case 4

The above four cases have been described in full detail elsewhere. [39]

It is quite obvious from the above case studies that MTH-68/H virus therapy is successful. The normal survival time for patients diagnosed with glioblastoma multiforme rarely exceeds more than one year; this diagnosis often spells a death sentence. However, with the MTH-68/H virus therapy, patients diagnosed with glioblastoma are far exceeding these limited time frames. During the long time of survival a malignization (immunophenotype changes) of glial tumors cannot be ascertained. A great majority of patients with glioblastomas live a very limited, bed-ridden life that is far from their daily routine. Because of the MTH-68/H virus therapy, the patients described had in fact returned to living a far more normal life, resuming many of their usual daily activities and way of living. From the case studies, it should also be duly noted that our group (Csatary and co-workers) have maintained use of the virus therapy over a long period of time, with some of the patients taking the therapy for years at a time. The possible secret behind the success of the therapy is that the viral therapy is continuously administered over a long period of time.

Since 1996, when MTH-68/H viral treatment was extended to high-grade gliomas, altogether 13 patients (including the above 4 patients) suffering from such tumors have been treated. In 6 patients the treatment did not arrest tumor growth, they died of the progression of their neoplasm. Two patients died of causes unrelated to their brain tumor. Two patients died after first responding favorably to MTH-68/H therapy. One of these is included here as Case 3, the other is not included here, but will be the subject of an in-depth analysis of the patient's clinical course in a future publication. The four patients described have exhibited survival times between 6 to 10 years post beginning viral treatment and offer reliable grounds to demonstrate the efficacy of oncolytic viral treatment. All four patients described in this writing had exhausted the potentials of conventional therapeutic modalities and were in the phase of relentless progression of their tumor, when beginning MTH-68/H therapy. There are additionally a limited number of individual glioma patients, who are presently under MTH-68/H therapy, a few demonstrating significant clinical improvement, but their survival times are still not long enough to allow for full evaluation.

Discussion

In the four cases of GBM and anaplastic astrocytomas reported by us in this case study, each of the four patients had the MTH-68/H virus therapy administered after the three anti-neoplastic classical modalities had been exhausted. This therapy was given to them for a longer period of time, much longer than other researchers have done with other viral therapies. Moreover, our definition of survival differs from others and is not simply living, but rather incorporates the idea that these patients return to their previous daily routines, to a more normal way of living. These patients have truly shown great clinical improvement.

Similar results have also been found in other human neoplasms and have been published. [32,34]

It is quite possible that some authors would attempt to interpret our results as a form of spontaneous regression (SR). Spontaneous regression is defined as an occurrence when the malignant neoplastic mass partially or completely disappears without any treatment or as a result of therapy considered inadequate to influence systemic neoplastic disease. [40,41] This definition is accepted, but it should be noted that the true existence of SR of neoplasms is often questioned and some simply do not accept this pathophysiological phenomenon. SR was reported in a case of pilocytic astrocytoma in a patient without neurofibromatosis type 1, but never in high grade glial tumors. [43] The employment of an oncolytic virus therapy is a very specific alternative and in part immunotherapeutic anti-neoplastic treatment.

Neoplasm associated markers (NAMs) are the biochemical and immunological counterparts of the morphology of neoplasms. [43,44] The expression of an immunocytochemically defined cell adhesion molecule (CAM) is also related to the tissue of origin and is not a random event.

During the past two decades, the use of monoclonal antibodies (MoABs) against oncofetal, neoplasm associated, cell lineage specific, differentiation, cancer/testis, endothelial, and cell proliferation related antigens in the diagnosis, biological assessment of prognosis, and in the immunotherapy of systematic neoplastic disease has gained increased importance. [45] A sensitive direct correlation exists between the expression of certain molecules and the development of an invasive, highly malignant cellular immunophenotype (CIP) of neoplastic cells, allowing for the occurrence of angiogenesis and metastasis. The development of molecular biological neoplasm detection has led to the development of different neoplasm associated antigens (NAAs). NAAs have been used in the immuno-diagnostic of human malignancies and in various neoplasms as immunotherapy through monoclonal antibodies. In the case of brain tumors, however, such protocols of using MoABs has never been established and has, thus far, proven to be unsuccessful.

The MTH-68/H virus therapy is three decades in the making, with the pioneering work of one of our group, (L.K.Cs) beginning his initial work using this therapy over three decades ago. [19] In the last five years, there are several clinical trials beginning employing other NDV oncolytic strains as virus onco-therapy, with some encouraging preliminary results. Clinical trials are planned using MTH-68/H, in the diagnosis of high grade gliomas. The MTH-68/H viral therapy has only been employed once the other classical anti-neoplastic treatments have failed and it has, nonetheless, achieved great success. How many more decades of results are needed for this therapy to be accepted as a permanent treatment modality of human neoplasms, especially since this therapy does not interfere with the three classical modalities and can potentially actually enhance the therapeutic effects of these already accepted treatments?

References

[1] Virchow, R. *Cellular pathology.* (RM de Witt, New York, 1860).

[2] Bodey B., Bodey B. Jr., and Siegel S.E. Immunophenotypical (IP) differential diagnosis and immunobiology of childhood primary brain tumors. A decade of experience. *Int J Pediatric Hematol/Oncol 6*, 65-84 (1998).

[3] von Deimling, A., Louis, D.N., and Wiestler, O.D. Molecular pathways in the formation of gliomas. *Glia 15*, 328-338 (1995).

[4] Kleihues, P., Soylemezoglu, F., Schauble, B., Scheithauer, B.W., and Burger, P.C. Histopathology, classification, and grading of gliomas. *Glia 15*, 211-221 (1995).

[5] Williams, B.P., Abney, E.R., and Raff, M.C. Macroglial cell development in embryonic rat brain: studies using monoclonal antibodies, fluorescence-activated cell sorting and cell culture. *Dev Biol 112*, 126-134 (1985).

[6] Katsura, S., Suzuki, J., and Wada, T. Statistical study of brain tumours in the neurosurgical clinics in Japan. *J Neurosurg 16*, 570-580 (1959).

[7] Cairncross, J.G. The biology of astrocytoma: lessons learned from chronic myelogenous leukemia-hypothesis. *J Neuro-Oncol 5*, 99-104 (1987).

[8] Greaves, M., Janossy, G., Francis, G., and Minowada, J. Membrane phenotypes of human leukemic cells and leukemic cell lines: Clinical correlates and biological implications. In: Differentiation of normal and neoplastic hemopoietic cells. Vol. 5 (Clarkson B, Marks PL, and Till J, eds) 823-841 (Cold Spring Harbor Conferences on Cell Proliferation, Cold Spring Harbor Laboratory, New York, 1977).

[9] Burns, B.F. Molecular genetic markers in lymphoproliferative disorders. *Clin Biochem 22*, 33-39 (1989).

[10] Bodey, B., Zeltzer, P.M., Saldivar, V., and Kemshead, J.: Immunophenotyping of childhood astrocytomas with a library of monoclonal antibodies. *Int J Cancer 45*, 1079-1087 (1990).

[11] Bullard, D.E., Gillespie, Y., Mahaley, M.S., and Bigner, D.D. Immunobiology of human gliomas. *Semin Oncol 13*, 94-109 (1986).

[12] Ohgaki, K., Schäuble, B., zur Hausen, A., von Ammon, K., and Kleihues, P. Genetic alterations associated with the evolution and progression of astrocytic brain tumors. *Virchows Arch 427*, 113-118 (1995).

[13] Bodey, B., Gröger, A.M., Bodey, B. Jr., Siegel, S.E., and Kaiser, H.E. Immunocytochemical detection of p53 protein expression in various childhood astrocytoma subtypes: Significance in tumor progression. *Anticancer Research 17*, 1187-1194 (1997).

[14] Biernat, W., Kleihues, P., Yonekawa, Y., and Ohgaki, H. Amplification and overexpression of MDM2 in primary (de novo) glioblastomas. *J Neuropathol Exp Neurol 56*, 180-185 (1997).

[15] Watanabe, K. *et al.* Overexpression of the EGF receptor and p53 mutations are mutually exclusive in the evolution of primary and secondary glioblastomas. *Brain Pathol 6*, 217-223 (1996).

[16] Watanabe, K., Tachibana, O., Yonekawa, Y., Kleihues, P., and Ohgaki, H. Role of gemistocytes in astrocytoma progression. *Lab Invest 76*, 277-284 (1997).

[17] Pollack, I.F., Campbell, J.W., Hamilton, R.L., Martinez, A.J., and Bozik, M.E: Proliferation index as a predictor of prognosis in malignant gliomas of childhood. *Cancer 79*, 849-856 (1997).

[18] Jay, V., Edwards, V., Halliday, W., Rutka, J., and Lau, R. "Polyphenotypic" tumors in the central nervous system: problems in nosology and classification. *Pediatr Pathol Lab Med 17*, 369-389 (1997).

[19] Csatary, L.K. Viruses in the treatment of cancer. *Lancet 2*, 825 (1971).

[20] Csatary, L.K., Romvary, J., Kasza, L., Schaff, S., and Massey, R.J. *In vivo* interference between pathogenic and non-pathogenic viruses. *J Med 16*, 563-573 (1985).

[21] Webb, H.E., and Gordon-Smith, C.E. Viruses in the treatment of cancer. *Lancet 1*, 1206-1208 (1970).

[22] Cassell, W., and Garrett, R.E.: Newcastle disease virus as an antineoplastic agent. *Cancer 18*, 863-868 (1965).

[23] Csatary, L.K. *et al.* Attenuated veterinary virus vaccine for the treatment of cancer. *Cancer Detection and Prevention 17*, 619-627 (1993).

[24] Csatary, L.K., Csatary, E., and Moss, R.W. Re: Scientific interest in Newcastle Disease Virus is reviving. *J Natl Cancer Inst 92*, 493-494 (2000).

[25] Walker, P.R., and Sikorska, M.: New aspects of the mechanism of DNA fragmentation in apoptosis. *Biochem Cell Biol 75:* 287-299, 1997.

[26] Walker, P.R., Saas, P., and Dietrich, P-Y. Role of Fas ligand (CD95L) in immune escape: the tumor cells strikes back. *J Immunol 158*, 4521-4524 (1997).

[27] Mule, J.J., Schwarz, S.L., Roberts, A.B., Sporn, M.B., and Rosenberg, S.A. Transforming growth factor-beta inhibits the *in vitro* generation of lymphokine-activated killer cells and cytotoxic T cells. *Cancer Immunol Immunother 26*, 95-100 (1988).

[28] Sporn, M.B., Roberts, A.B., Wakefield, L.M., and Assoian, R.K. Transforming growth factor-beta: biological function and chemical structure. *Science 233*, 532-534 (1986).

[29] Rivoltini, L., *et al.* Phenotypic and functional analysis of lymphocytes infiltrating paediatric tumours, with a characterization of the tumour phenotype. *Cancer Immunol Immunother 34*, 241-251 (1992).

[30] Bodey B., Bodey B. Jr., and Siegel S.E. Immunophenotypic characterization of infiltrating poly- and mononuclear cells in childhood brain tumors. *Modern Pathology 8*, 333-338 (1995).

[31] Bodey B., Bodey B. Jr., Siegel S.E., and Kaiser H.E. Immunocytochemical detection of leukocyte-associated and apoptosis-related antigen expression in childhood brain tumors. *Critical Reviews Oncology/Hematology 39*, 3-16 (2001).

[32] Csatary, L.K., *et al.*: Beneficial treatment of patients with advanced cancer using a Newcastle disease virus vaccine (MTH-68/H). *Anticancer Res 19*, 635-638 (1999).

[33] Csatary LK. et al. Use of Newcastle Disease Virus Vaccine (MTH-68/H) in a Patient With High-grade Glioblastoma; *JAMA,* May 5, 1999. Vol 281, No *17* pp 1588-1589.

[34] Csatary, LK, et al. ,Treatment of Malignant Tumors with Attenuated Newcastle Disease Virus Vaccine; A Phase II Trial, *Lege Artis Medicinae*, *4(7)* pp 640- 645, 1994.

[35] Ballagi-Pordány et al., Identification and grouping of Newcastle disease virus strains by restriction site analysis of a region from the F gene, *Archives of Virology*, *141*, 243-261.,1996.

[36] Sakaguchi T., Newcastle disease virus evolution. I. Multiple lineages defined by sequence variability of the hemagglutinin-neuraminidase gene. *Virology 169*: 260-272, 1989.

[37] Fábián, Zs., Torocsik B, Csatary L.K, Kiss K, Szeberenyi J.. Induction of apoptosis by a Newcastle Disease Virus vaccine (MTH-68/H) in PC12 rat phaeochromocytoma cells. *Anticancer Research 21*, 125-135 (2001).

[38] Szeberényi J., Fabian Zs., Torocsik B, Kiss K, Csatary, LK; Newcastle Disease Virus Induced Apoptosis in PC12 Phaeochromosytoma Cells, *Amer. J. Therapeutics 10 (4):* 282-8, 2003.

[39] Csatary LK., Gosztonyi G., Liszka V., Bodey B., Csatary CM.; MTH-68/H Oncolytic Viral Treatment in Human High-Grade Gliomas *Journal of Neuro-Oncology*, *67*: 83-93, 2004

[40] Bodey B., Bodey B. Jr., Siegel S.E., and Kaiser H.E. Spontaneous regression of neoplasms in mammals. Review of the cases published between 1988 and 1997. *IN VIVO 12*, 107-122 (1998).

[41] Bodey B. Spontaneous Regression of Neoplasms: New Possibilities for Immunotherapy. *EOBT*, in print (2002).

[42] 42.. Gallucci, M., Catalucci, A., Scheithauer, B.W., and Forbes G.S. Spontaneous involution of pilocytic astrocytoma in a patient without neurofibromatosis type 1: case report. *Radiology 214*, 223-226 (2000).

[43] Bodey, B. The significance of immunocytochemistry in the diagnosis and therapy of neoplasms. *EOBT 2*, 371-393 (2002).

[44] Bodey B., Bodey B. Jr, Siegel S.E., and Kaiser H.E. Fas (APO-1, CD95) receptor expression in childhood astrocytomas. Is it a marker of the major apoptotic pathway or a signaling receptor for immune escape of neoplastic cells? *IN VIVO 13*, 357-373 (1999).

[45] Bodey B. Genetically Engineered Antibodies for Direct Anti-Neoplastic Treatment and Neoplastic Cells Directed Delivery of Various Therapeutic Agents. *EOBT 1*, 603-617 (2001).

In: Focus on Brain Cancer Research
Editor: Andrew V. Yang, pp. 83-98
ISBN 1-59454-973-7

Chapter V

Review of Genetic Mutations of Gliomas in the Malay Population and its Reflections of Tumorigenesis in South East Asia

***J. Abdullah*[*1], *M. Mohd Ghazali*[1], *K. Asmarina*[1], *A. Farizan*[1], *N. M Isa*[2] and *H. Jaafar*[3]**

[1]Department of Neurosciences, [2] Human Genome Center, [3]Department of Pathology, School of Medical Sciences, Universiti Sains Malaysia, Kubang Kerian, Kelantan, Malaysia.

Abstract

Gliomas are the most common type of primary malignant brain tumors in Malaysia. Several ideas have emerged about the genetic alterations occurring in human cancers and how they contribute to tumorigenesis. The role of common genetic alterations in determining the range of individual susceptibility within the population are being increasingly recognized. The accumulation of genetic alterations are thought to drive the progression of normal cells through hyperplastic and dysplastic stages to invasive cancer and, finally, metastatic disease. With regards to that, numerous research have been aggressively carried out, focusing on the potential roles of genes which are important in cell cycle progression as well as apoptotic pathways. The results revealed *PTEN* and *p53* genes mutations to be found in mostly high grade gliomas. Loss of heterozygosity (LOH) and telomerase activities were also found in high grade glioma cases, suggesting that those actions might contribute to brain tumorigenesis in Malaysia especially amongst the

* Corresponding Author: Professor Dr. Jafri Malin Abdullah, Department of Neurosciences, School of Medical Sciences, University Science Malaysia, 16150 Kubang Kerian, Kelantan, Malaysia. Tel: +609-7664240. Fax: +609-7648613. Email address: deptneurosciencesppspusm@yahoo.com.

Malay population. The identification of genes and pathways involved would enhance our understanding of the biology of this process. It would also provide new targets for early diagnosis and facilitate treatment design for example in developing DNA vaccine as an anti-cancer agent and virus therapy which has shown promise as a cancer treatment in Malaysia.

Introduction

Abnormal proliferation, inability of cells to die and their potential to modify their tissue environment results from accumulation of genetic aberrations [1]. The development of an invasive brain tumor involves a multistep process that has been associated with the altered expression of several oncogenes and tumor-suppressor genes. Advances in molecular biology in the past decades have revolutionized our understanding of cancer, including brain tumors. The detailed understanding of molecular events responsible for brain tumor will lead to the development of better techniques for the diagnosis and classification of human brain as well as the ultimate goal of rationally based therapy [2, 3]

A total of 21,464 cancer cases were diagnosed among Malaysians in Peninsular Malaysia in the year 2003, comprising 9,400 males and 12,064 females. A significant proportion of central nervous system neoplasms affects children in Malaysia, ranked second in incidence after leukemias with the cancer incidence per 100,000 population of 1.7 in male and 1.6 in female [4]. Gliomas are tumors of neuroepithelial origin and include the type of astrocytic tumors, oligodendroglial tumors, mixed gliomas, ependymomas and neuroepithelial tumors of uncertain origin [5]. It is the most common type of brain tumors, constituting more than 50% of all brain tumors and 2% of the malignant tumors in adults [6]. Astrocytic tumors occur in only 25% of patients in Singapore with primary brain tumors [7]. In gliomas, molecular genetic analyses play an increasing part in the classification and the treatment planning. As the largest and most important group of brain tumors, they have been receiving considerable attention from cancer geneticists.

PTEN and LOH in Glioma Cases

Among the frequently reported cases in molecular genetic research of brain tumors, *PTEN* mutations and Loss of Heterozygosity (LOH) have been suggested to play significant roles in the poor prognosis of the cancer.

In gliomas, *PTEN* gene abnormalities are preferentially found in high-grade gliomas, particularly in glioblastoma multiforme [8-12]. Deletions of the *PTEN* region at 10q23 are also reported as predominant findings in glioblastoma [11, 13, 14]. *PTEN* alterations are detectable in a low fraction (<10%) of anaplastic astrocytomas and anaplastic oligodendrogliomas and when present, indicate a poor prognosis [15].

Though association of LOH in brain tumors is not strongly correlated, frequent of allelic losses were reported in malignant astrocytoma, glioblastoma, anaplastic oligodendroglioma and ependymoma cases. In malignant astrocytoma, regular of allelic losses were defined in chromosome 10, 13q, 17p and 22q, suggesting the presence of tumor suppressor genes on this chromosomes [16]. They have also reported the LOH cases on chromosome 17p in anaplastic oligodendroglioma samples. LOH on chromosome 10 and 13q [16] were found in most anaplastic ependymoma cases. While in glioblastomas, with partial loss of chromosome 10, at least three common deletions were found which were 10q14-pter, 10q23-24 and 10q25-qter, suggestive of multiple tumor suppressor genes [17]. Forty to 60% of reported deletion in glioblastoma cases occurred on chromosome 9p21 [18].

Several studies have shown that loss of heterozygosity as well as *PTEN* mutation were correlated with poor prognosis in glioma patients [19]. They suggested that by losing function of those regions, the survival rates of the patients decreased. In our study, we found that *PTEN* mutations are infrequently reported among Malay patients. However, results showed that 21.6% of the reported *PTEN* mutations were mostly found in high grade of glioma cases [20]. Additionally, LOH was frequently occurring among Malay high grade glioma patients where 32.4% LOH was detected. Univariate Cox regression analysis revealed that histopathological grade, vascularity, *PTEN*, LOH and combined presence of *PTEN* and LOH were significant prognostic factors for the survival of patients with brain tumor in Malaysia. However, multivariate analyses indicate that no single variable was the prognostic factor for the survival [12].

Telomerase Activity with Undetectable *p16* Gene Mutation in Glioma

Another tumor suppressor gene which is frequently implicated in tumorigenesis is *p16 (MTS1/CDKN2A/INK4A)* which is located on chromosome 9p21, which plays a major role in regulating the cell cycle at the G1–S check point. The *p16* gene was firstly demonstrated by Kamb, *et al.* in 1994. This gene composed of three exons, which encodes a 156 amino acid, 15.8-kD protein that blocks progression of cell cycle, so indirectly prevent cells from entering into the S phase through the G1 phase [22, 23]. Loss of this protein function may lead to cancer progression by allowing unregulated cellular proliferation [22].

The important role of *p16* gene in the occurrence of many types of cancer was first suggested by high frequent mutations and deletions of this gene in human cancer cell lines. Alterations of the *p16* gene are known to occur in many primary tumors through different mechanisms including homozygous deletion, point mutation, and hypermethylation of the *p16* gene promoter. PCR-SSCP (Single Strand Conformation Polymorphism) analysis was performed to screen for *p16* gene mutation at exon 1 and 2. There was no mobility shift of *p16* gene using SSCP with no mutations at exon 1 and 2 in all samples. These results suggest that another mechanism of *p16* gene alterations could be involved [20].

Recent studies have shown that activation of the telomerase is necessary for tumorigenesis. The length of the telomeres decreases due to the end replication problem with every cell division. This problem can be prevented by maintaining telomeric length. Both telomerase and telomere have been identified as targets for anticancer therapy since there were evidences of strong correlations between telomerase reactivation, cellular immortalization and cancer [24].

We detected 6 out of 23 cases (26.1%) of telomerase activities in our brain tumor samples which mostly presented as high-grade tumors. We determined telomerase activity in 23 tumor tissues base on the PCR-Telomeric Repeat Amplification Protocol (TRAP) assay using $TRAP_{EZE}$ Telomerase Detection Kit (Intergen Co., USA). Previous studies have reported similar findings of telomerase activities in glioblastoma multiforme, oligodendroglioma and medulloblastoma [25, 26]. There was a significant association between telomerase activity status and tumor grade but not with patient criteria. Telomerase activity was detected in the analyzed tumors, supporting the fact that activation of telomerase is an important feature for tumorigenesis.

p53

An important prognostic factor in gliomas is the status of the *p53* tumor-suppressor gene in the primary tumor.Alteration of the tumor suppressor gene *p53* is considered to be a critical step in the development of human cancer. It is located on chromosome 17p and has been found to influence multiple cellular functions, including progression through the cell cycle, DNA repair after radiation damage, genomic stability and also induces G1 arrest or apoptosis in a cell-type-dependent manner via the upregulation of another CDK inhibitor, *p21/WAF1.18* [27, 28].

Changes in this gene have been detected in a wide range of human tumors including gliomas and seem to be almost ubiquitous in human tumorigenesis [29]. In gliomas, the presence of *p53* gene alterations has been associated with worse prognosis. The *p53* gene often shows missense mutations in one allele and is found within exons 5 to 8 spanning the evolutionary conserved region of the protein in gliomas [30].

Forty-seven Malaysian glioma samples were analyzed using SSCP that showed *p53* mutations in 12 tumors with an incidence rate of 25.5%. Mutations were found in 2 patients of grade II, and 5 patients both in grade III and grade IV. The sequencing results revealed the presence of base-substitutions and frameshifts mutations in these glioma samples [31].

The 3 factors associated with *p53* mutations were grade, site and consistency of tumor by using univariate analysis, although multivariate analysis revealed no positive on predictors of mutation. As a conclusion although *p53* genetic alterations were involved in glioma patients in Malaysia, it has no impact on prognosis [31]. These results support the study that had been done by researchers in Singapore [7].

p27 Gene

p27 (kip1/*p27*kip1) is one of the cyclin-dependent kinase inhibitor (CDKI), which also plays important roles as a negative regulator in cell cycles [32, 33]. *p27* is encoded by CDKN1B gene, which is located on chromosome 12q13. The gene consists of three exons and is encoded for 4.99 kb of DNA.

In cell cycles, *p27* acts by binding to the cyclin-CDK complexes and inhibit their activities [34]. This disrupts the progression of G1 to S phase and leads to apoptosis of the cells [35].

Milas *et al.* (2002) reported that *p27* protein expression shows reduction after radiotherapy treatment. This was observed in several cancer cases. The same phenomenon had been identified in brain tumor cases, where a low level of *p27* protein expression during tumor progression was observed [37].

Alteration in CDKN1B gene may also contribute to dysfunction of *p27* as a tumor suppressor gene in controlling cell growth. These changes might have effect normal function and expression of the gene and increase the risk of tumor development [35]

p27 mutation was firstly reported by Morosetti *et al.* (1995). Throughout their research, they found non-sense mutation at codon 76 in adult T-lymphoma cases and homozygus deletion on exon 2 in B-immunoblastic lymphoma cases. Related to that, they suggested that *p27* mutation might have an important role in those tumor progresion. In 1996, Spirin *et al.* reported other mutations of *p27* in breast cancer. They found 2 types of mutation, a polymorphism at codon 142 and a non-sense mutation at codon 104.

Research in Malaysia found no alteration of *p27* gene in Malay glioma patients [40]. The result showed that *p27* gene alteration might have not contributed much to the development of glioma cases in Malaysia.

Cyclin D1 Gene

Cyclin D1 encoded by *CCND1* gene and located on chromosome 11q3 [41, 42]. *CCND1* consists of 5 exons, which encodes for 259 amino acids. *CCND1* is also known as *PRAD1, Cyl-1, Bcl-1, U21B31, D11S287E* AND hgnc: 988 (Human Nomenclature Databases).

Cyclin D1 is classified as one of the proto-oncogen [42, 43] and is frequently associated with tumor development. Cyclin D1 protein overexpresion are frequently reported in most cancer cases including brain tumors. High level of Cyclin D1 expression will cause shortage in G1 phase and induce progression of G1 phase to S phase in cell cycles.

There are some studies done on Cyclin D1 protein overexpression and some researchers suggested that this phenomenon occurs as a result of gene amplification [44, 45]. Cyclin D1 gene amplification have frequently been suggested to contribute to the development of many cancer types including head and neck squamous cell carcinoma, cervical carcinoma and oral squamous cell carcinoma [45, 46].

Nishimoto *et al* (2004) have reported that Cyclin D1 gene polymorphism also plays important roles in the development of squamous cell carcinoma of the upper aerodigestive tract. Another study carried out by Kong *et al* (2000) found that Cyclin D1 gene polymorphism effected the age of onset of Hereditary nonpolyposis colorectal cancer.

Findings by Moreno-Bueno *et al.* (2003) proposed that mutation of *CCND1* is one of the unreported mechanisms, which also contribute to Cyclin D1 overexpression. They found that 12 bp of *CCND1* gene was deleted in endometrial cancer and they predicted this as another pathway to contribute to the development of the cancer.

Research carried out in Malaysia with the purpose of studying the role of Cyclin D1 gene in brain tumorigenesis found only one (9%) G base deletion in Malay glioma cases, suggesting that Cyclin D1 gene alteration is infrequent in the Malay population. However, the alteration of Cyclin D1 gene might play important roles in brain tumorigenesis. Base deletion of Cyclin D1 gene will lead to formation of abnormal protein which in turn, may cause cells to proliferate uncontrollably [40].

Mutation in Pro-Apoptotic Gene *Bax*

Apoptosis is an inter-related collection of pathways and mechanisms utilized to eliminate excess or unwanted cells, including neurons, in the developmental stages [50]. Pathologic roles have been defined in cancer biology. Tumor cells that inhibit apoptosis show a growth advantage over normal tissue [51]. One of the principal death-signaling pathways involves the mitochondrion, which acts by stabilizing mitochondrial function and suppressing the release of cytochrome c [52, 53]. The study of apoptosis is relevant to many aspects of cancer biology, which include tumorigenesis, tumor homeostasis, angiogenesis, metastasis and clinical treatment [54].

Bax is a strong pro-apoptotic gene that induces apoptosis, which is located on chromosome 19. It consists of six exons and a promoter region. The authors of numerous studies have attempted to address whether the mutation of *Bax* gene has a prognostic role in patients with tumors. Sequence variations in the promoter region and the coding sequence can abolish its pro-apoptotic function [55]. Mutation of *Bax* gene is also an important mechanism for loss of Bax expression. The *Bax* gene mutation has been suggested to play an important role in endometrial, gastric and colorectal cancers. It also has been considered as a potential tumor suppressor.[56]

In determining the potential of genetic variation in gliomas we analyzed mutation in exon 6 of *Bax* gene. Our results showed genetic alterations in 5% of our glioma sample for *Bax* gene. The alteration occurred at nucleotide 153 of *Bax* gene which resulted in C base deletion [57]. This might cause loss of Bax expression and will further enhance the escape of tumor cells from apoptotic cell death and promote malignant progression of the tumor cells.

Matrix Metalloproteinase-3 Gene Variation

Matrix Metalloproteinases (MMPs) are the largest group of extracellular matrix-degrading enzymes and so far 22 members have been found in human tissue [58]. MMPs are a family of closely related, metal-dependent endopeptidases. Once activated, MMPs will degrade a variety of extracellular matrix and basement membrane components [59, 60].

MMP family has substrate-specific degradation activity. Specifically, Matrix Metalloproteinse-3 (MMP-3) acts on type IV collagen that forms basal membrane [61]. Expression of most MMPs is normally low in tissues and is induced when remodelling of extracellular matrix is required. Numerous studies have shown that a high expression of MMPs in brain tumors is correlated with an increased aggressiveness of tumors.

Recently, a naturally occurring sequence variation in the human *MMP-3* gene promoter has been reported [62]. *MMP-3* gene maps on chromosome 11, at 11q22.3. *MMP-3* gene encoded Matrix metalloproteinase-3 which also known as stromelysin 1 or progelatinase. Changes in MMP-3 biosynthesis usually proceed with changes in gene transcription and at the mRNA level. The insertion of an A in the *MMP-3* gene promoter sequence halves its transcription activity.

It has been described that there are functional polymorphism at position –1171 bp upstream from the start of the transcription of promoter sequence *MMP-3* gene, consisting in a stretch of five or six adenosines [63]. In vitro assays of promoter activity showed that 5A allele had 2-fold higher promoter activity than the 6A allele. The polymorphism that has been recently tested would enhance cancers susceptibility in lymphatic metastasis of non-small cell lung carcinoma, renal cell carcinoma, breast, ovarian and colorectal cancer [62, 64-66]. It was, however, unclear whether the 5A/6A polymorphism plays a role in the regulation of stromelysin-1 expression in gliomas. Our study showed those 5A alleles were detected in more than 80% of our glioma samples [67].

ras, c-myc and EGFR

ras gene families consists of 3 members: *N-ras, H-ras* and *K-ras,* which encodes for the highly homologous protein so called p21 according to their molecular weight. The inactivation of *ras* gene by point mutation are the most frequent and it is well known that in genetics an alteration can be associated with human cancers including brain tumors. Common mechanisms of inactivation of these genes are missense mutations at the well known hot spot codon 12, 13 and 16 [68]. Activating point mutations have been localized in codons 12, 13, 59, 61, 63, 116,117, 119 and 146 [69]. All these alterations occur at or near the guanine nucleotide biding sites.

The presence of *ras* mutation has also been shown to be significant in terms of prognosis. Considering it's importance, the *ras* gene might be the good target for the development of anticancer therapy [70]. Our results revealed that no ras mutations were present when using PCR-SSCP analyses in the DNA extracted from our gliomas tissues.

According to Yusoff et al (2004), Zan et al (2003) and Ghazali et al (2005), there were no *ras* mutations detected in all tumour analyzed from Malaysian patients [71-73]. They concluded that these genes did not play a major role in tumourgenesis mainly in malignant gliomas. A previous study which involved direct sequencing analysis in oral tumours also reported that no mutation were found in *N-ras, K-ras* and *H-ras* genes [74]. Activating *ras* mutations can be found in human malignancies with an overall frequency of 15-20%. A high incidence of *ras* gene mutations has been reported in malignant tumors of the pancreas (80-90%, *K-ras*), in colorectal carcinomas (30-60%), in non-melanoma skin cancer (30-50%, *H-ras*), in hematopoietic neoplasia of myeloid origin (18-30%, *K*-and *N-ras*) and in seminoma (25-40%, *K-ras*) [75]. In other tumors, a mutant *ras* gene is found at a lower frequency: in breast carcinoma (0-12%, *K-ras*), glioblastoma and neuroblastoma (0-10%, *K-* and *N-ras*) (69].

The *c-myc* gene was discovered as the cellular homolog of the retroviral v-myc oncogene 20 years ago [76, 77]. The c-myc proto-oncogene was subsequently found to be activated in various animal and human tumors [78-80]. It belonged to the family of *myc* gene that included *B-myc, L-myc, N-myc* and *s-myc*; however only *c-myc, L-myc* and *N-myc* have had neoplastic potential [81].

The *c-myc* gene, mapped on human chromosome 8q24, encodes the transcription factor c-myc, which heterodimerizes with a partner protein, Max, to regulate gene expression. The amplification of the *n-myc* gene in neuroblastomas appears to correlate with the clinical stage of the tumor and with the poor prognosis of the patients. Therefore it is tempting to speculate that the n-myc protein is one of the essential products necessary for the aberrant behavior of neuroblastoma cells [82].

c-myc's status as an important target was reinforced by a recent widely-reported paper published in Science by Dean Felsher at Stanford, in which he demonstrated that a temporary reduction in c-Myc expression followed by reactivation, in a genetically engineered mouse model, induced highly selective and complete apoptosis in cancer cells, while having no effect on normal cells [83].

In human cancers, the *c-myc* gene is activated through several mechanisms. Investigation of *c-myc* gene alterations in glioma may provide important knowledge about the genetic basis which is based on fact that alteration in *c-myc* gene may contribute to the overexpression and amplification of c-myc [84]. The frequency of genetic alterations of *c-myc* gene in human cancer [80] has allowed estimation that approximately 70,000 US cancer deaths per year are associated with changes in the c-myc gene or its expression. C-myc may contribute to one-seventh of US cancer deaths, recent efforts have been directed towards understanding the function of the c-myc protein in cancer biology with the hope that therapeutic insights will emerge [76, 85, 86]. The *c-myc* gene is amplified in various human cancers such as lung carcinoma [87], breast carcinoma [88] and rare cases of colon carcinoma [89]. Ghazali et al (2005) showed that no abnormal migration shifts were detected in the entire glioma sample analyzed for mutation on *c-myc* gene in North East Malaysian patients using the PCR-SSCP technique [86].

Molecular abnormalities associated with primary brain tumors include a wide variety of changes in tumor suppressor gene, proto-oncogenes and growth factors. The *EGFR* gene is a multifocal allosteric transmembrane protein with an intra cellular binding site for EGF, and acts as a tyrosine kinase. The gene is localized on the short arm of chromosome 7, within 7p11 – 13, and is called erb – B1. This receptor has been found to be over-expressed in 50% to 70% of glioblastoma multiforme. Although the functions of the proteins encoded by the most proto-oncogenes are not precisely known, biochemical activities of several proto-oncogene products have been identified. Some of the gene products are identical or related to, proteins, known to be important in growth regulation.

The current interests of molecular abnormalities in brain tumours have led our group to study *EGFR* gene mutation in relation to gliomas occurrence. In determining the genetic variations in *EGFR* genes, glioma samples were subjected to polymerase chain reaction (PCR). Amplified products were then directly sequenced. The results revealed no *EGFR* gene alterations were found in all of our glioma samples.

According to a the previous study, *EGFR* gene was often mutated in high-grade gliomas in adults, but the frequency of EGFR mutations was still low. Ghazali et al (2005) indicated that there was no alteration of *EGFR* gene via PCR-SSCP and point mutation in exon 1 from Malaysian patients and this gene might not play a major role in tumourigenesis [86]. David et al found that *EGFR* gene amplifications does not occur in Pleomorphic xanthoastrocytoma (PXA) but glioblastoma multiformee (GBM) that arise from PXA may display *EGFR* gene amplification. In adult gangliogliomas, another benign form of astrocytic glioma, *EGFR* gene amplification or allelic loss on chromosomes 10, 13q, 17p, 19q and 22q was not detected.

In simple logistic regression analysis of all three genes analyzed where there were no alteration of ras, c-myc and EGFR, clinical and radiological variables which were found to be significant were hemiplegia (Crude OR 23.29, 95% CI 2.84- 225.45, p=0.004), vascularity (Crude OR = 5.5, 95% CI 1.03 – 29.48, p=0.047) and response to radiotherapy (Crude OR=13.75, 95% CI 2.47-76.42, p=0.003). For those who were hemiplegic, they were 25 times more likely to have a high pathological grade compared to those without hemiplegia. Patients with vascular involvement were 5.5 times more likely to have higher pathological grade. However, this finding was not significant in multivariate analysis. Patients who had radiotherapy were nearly 14 times more likely to have higher pathological grade.

Multivariate analysis revealed that patients with hemiplegia were more likely to have higher pathological grade (adjusted OR =171.36, 95% CI 388 – 7566.01, p= 0.008). For those who had higher pathological grading were 80 times more likely to have radiotherapy (adjusted OR 80.92, 95% CI 3.94-1662.91, p=0.004). Other variables were found as insignificant. Our Malaysian patients with malignant gliomas, studied with no ras, c-myc and EGFR mutations, are still alive 6 years after treatment.

Conclusion and Future Directions

Multiple genetic alterations are sequentially occurring in carcinogenesis of many cancer types including brain tumors. Many of the abnormalities usually lead to the loss of normal progress through cell cycle and overexpression of growth factors and/or their receptors. In addition, a number of genetic abnormalities have been listed, where the alterations of the markers are hopefully bringing new information on value of prognostication towards the patient's response to treatment.

Based on a cancer survey in Malaysia, brain tumors are the second most frequently reported cases, after leukaemia in children. The adult brain tumor cases are reported to have a crude increment of about 2000 new cases every year [90]. With regards to that, current research and findings are hopefully helpful in developing new approaches to treat brain tumors in Malaysian and South East Asian patients.

In recent years, gene therapy has become one of the most evolving therapeutic modality for malignant gliomas. With the neural stem cell-guided gene therapy, this approach could be significantly enhanced. *PTEN*, LOH and p53 could be among the targeted genes for therapy in malignant gliomas since those genes have showed frequent alterations among Malay patients and hopefully other South East Asian patients since the population is homogenously from the same anthropological stock. Besides that, a high frequency of telomerase activities in high grade gliomas patients were detected suggesting their importance in brain tumorigenesis. Antisense therapy for telomerase is one of the promising treatments which have been developed by a group of researchers [91] to inhibit human telomeric activities. Other malignant gliomas therapies which are being developed including oncolytic virus therapies [92, 93], angiogenesis inhibitor and neural stem cells. These are among the future promising approaches that could be universally applied.

Further investigations should be done to determine other brain tumor markers which could be useful for therapeutic purposes. This review opefully provides important knowledge of central nervous system tumour etiologies which are important for the development of prevention strategies. It is hope that more data will come out from South East Asian countries in the near future via a close and cohort collaboration.

Acknowledgement

We would like to acknowledge Majlis Kanser Nasional (MAKNA) for the grants supporting the studies of *c-Myc*, *Ras*, *EGFR*, *NF2*, *Bax*, *MMP-3*, *p27* and *Cyclin D1* genes, the short term grant under the Intensification of Research in Priority Areas (IRPA) for *PTEN* and LOH studies (No. 304/PPSP/6131122), FELDA Foundation for the support of *p16* and telomerase studies (No. 304/PPSP/6150033Y104), and The Malaysian Toray Research Foundation Grant for *p53* gene study (No. 380/0500/5051). We would also like to acknowledge Professor Mohd Nizam Isa who was directly involved in these IRPA projects until the year 2002.

References

[1] Santarius T, Kirsch M, Rossi ML, Black PM. Molecular aspects of neuro-oncology. *Clin Neurol Neurosurg* 1997;99(3):184-95.

[2] Michael D. Taylor KTJTR. Neurogenetics and the molecular biology of human brain tumors. In: JR AHKERL, editor. *Brain Tumors An encyclopaedic approach.* London: Churchill Livingstone; 2001. p. 71-103.

[3] Hilton DA, Melling C. Genetic markers in the assessment of intrinsic brain tumours. *Current Diagnostic Pathology* 2004;10: 83–92.

[4] Lim G, Halimah Y, editors. Second Report of the National Cancer Registry. Cancer Incidence in Malaysia 2003. 2 ed: National Cancer Registry. Kuala Lumpur; 2004.

[5] Kleihues P, Louis DN, Scheithauer BW, Rorke LB, Reifenberger G, Burger PC, et al. The WHO classification of tumors of the nervous system. *J Neuropathol Exp Neurol* 2002;61(3):215-25; discussion 226-9.

[6] Phatak P, Selvi SK, Divya T, Hegde AS, Hegde S, Somasundaram K. Alterations in tumour suppressor gene p53 in human gliomas from Indian patients. *J Biosci* 2002;27(7):673-8.

[7] Das A, Tan WL, Teo J, Smith DR. Glioblastoma multiformee in an Asian population: evidence for a distinct genetic pathway. *J Neurooncol* 2002;60(2):117-25.

[8] Davies MP, Gibbs FE, Halliwell N, Joyce KA, Roebuck MM, Rossi ML, et al. Mutation in the *PTEN*/MMAC1 gene in archival low grade and high grade gliomas. *Br J Cancer* 1999;79(9-10):1542-8.

[9] Hill JR, Kuriyama N, Kuriyama H, Israel MA. Molecular genetics of brain tumors. *Arch Neurol* 1999;56(4):439-41.

[10] Maier D, Zhang Z, Taylor E, Hamou MF, Gratzl O, Van Meir EG, et al. Somatic deletion mapping on chromosome 10 and sequence analysis of *PTEN*/MMAC1 point to the 10q25-26 region as the primary target in low-grade and high-grade gliomas. *Oncogene* 1998;16(25):3331-5.

[11] Rasheed BK, Stenzel TT, McLendon RE, Parsons R, Friedman AH, Friedman HS, et al. *PTEN* gene mutations are seen in high-grade but not in low-grade gliomas. *Cancer Res* 1997;57(19):4187-90.

[12] Zainuddin N, Jaafar H, Isa MN, Abdullah JM. Presence of allelic loss and *PTEN* mutations in malignant gliomas from Malay patients. *Med J Malaysia* 2004;59(4):468-79.

[13] Li J, Yen C, Liaw D, Podsypanina K, Bose S, Wang SI, et al. *PTEN*, a putative protein tyrosine phosphatase gene mutated in human brain, breast, and prostate cancer. *Science* 1997;275(5308):1943-7.

[14] Wang SI, Puc J, Li J, Bruce JN, Cairns P, Sidransky D, et al. Somatic mutations of *PTEN* in glioblastoma multiformee. *Cancer Res* 1997;57(19):4183-6.

[15] Knobbe CB, Merlo A, Reifenberger G. Pten signaling in gliomas. *Neuro-oncol* 2002;4(3):196-211.

[16] Lee SH, Kim JH, Rhee CH, Kang YS, Lee JH, Hong SI, et al. Loss of heterozygosity on chromosome 10, 13q(Rb), 17p, and p53 gene mutations in human brain gliomas. *J Korean Med Sci* 1995;10(6):442-8.

[17] Fujisawa H, Reis RM, Nakamura M, Colella S, Yonekawa Y, Kleihues P, et al. Loss of heterozygosity on chromosome 10 is more extensive in primary (de novo) than in secondary glioblastomas. *Lab Invest* 2000;80(1):65-72.

[18] Cheng Y, Ng HK, Ding M, Zhang SF, Pang JC, Lo KW. Molecular analysis of microdissected de novo glioblastomas and paired astrocytic tumors. *J Neuropathol Exp Neurol* 1999;58(2):120-8.

[19] Balesaria S, Brock C, Bower M, Clark J, Nicholson SK, Lewis P, et al. Loss of chromosome 10 is an independent prognostic factor in high-grade gliomas. *Br J Cancer* 1999;81(8):1371-7.

[20] Abdullah JM, Zainuddin N, Sulong S, Jaafar H, Isa MN. Molecular genetic analysis of phosphatase and tensin homolog and p16 tumor suppressor genes in patients with malignant glioma. *Neurosurg Focus* 2003;14(4):e6.

[21] Kamb A, Gruis NA, Weaver-Feldhaus J, Liu Q, Harshman K, Tavtigian SV, et al. A cell cycle regulator potentially involved in genesis of many tumor types. *Science* 1994;264(5157):436-40.

[22] Liggett WH, Jr., Sidransky D. Role of the p16 tumor suppressor gene in cancer. *J Clin Oncol* 1998;16(3):1197-206.

[23] Guang Z, Xianhou Y. Study of deletion of P16 gene in the progression of brain astrocytomas. *Chinese J Cancer Res* 1998;10:412-417.

[24] Urquidi V, Tarin D, Goodison S. Role of telomerase in cell senescence and oncogenesis. *Annu Rev Med* 2000;51:65-79.

[25] Chen HJ, Cho CL, Liang CL, Chen L, Chang HW, Lu K, et al. Differential telomerase expression and telomere length in primary intracranial tumors. *Chang Gung Med J* 2001;24(6):352-60.

[26] Sano T, Asai A, Mishima K, Fujimaki T, Kirino T. Telomerase activity in 144 brain tumours. *Br J Cancer* 1998;77(10):1633-7.

[27] Lane DP. Cancer. p53, guardian of the genome. *Nature* 1992;358(6381):15-6.

[28] Hussain SA, James ND. Molecular markers in bladder cancer. *Semin Radiat Oncol* 2005;15(1):3-9.

[29] Patt S, Gries H, Giraldo M, Cervos-Navarro J, Martin H, Janisch W, et al. p53 gene mutations in human astrocytic brain tumors including pilocytic astrocytomas. *Hum Pathol* 1996;27(6):586-9.

[30] Greenblatt MS, Bennett WP, Hollstein M, Harris CC. Mutations in the p53 tumor suppressor gene: clues to cancer etiology and molecular pathogenesis. *Cancer Res* 1994;54(18):4855-78.

[31] Yusoff AA, Abdullah J, Abdullah MR, Mohd Ariff AR, Isa MN. Association of p53 tumor suppressor gene with paraclinical and clinical modalities of gliomas patients in Malaysia. *Acta Neurochir* (Wien) 2004;146(6):595-601.

[32] Ferrando AA, Balbin M, Pendas AM, Vizoso F, Velasco G, Lopez-Otin C. Mutational analysis of the human cyclin-dependent kinase inhibitor *p27*kip1 in primary breast carcinomas. *Hum Genet* 1996;97(1):91-4.

[33] Shin JY, Kim HS, Lee KS, Kim J, Park JB, Won MH, et al. Mutation and expression of the *p27*KIP1 and p57KIP2 genes in human gastric cancer. *Exp Mol Med* 2000;32(2):79-83.

[34] Coqueret O. New roles for p21 and *p27* cell-cycle inhibitors: a function for each cell compartment? *Trends Cell Biol* 2003;13(2):65-70.

[35] Kang YK, Kim WH, Jang JJ. Expression of G1-S modulators (p53, p16, *p27*, cyclin D1, Rb) and Smad4/Dpc4 in intrahepatic cholangiocarcinoma. *Hum Pathol* 2002;33(9):877-83.

[36] Milas L, Akimoto T, Hunter NR, Mason KA, Buchmiller L, Yamakawa M, et al. Relationship between cyclin D1 expression and poor radioresponse of murine carcinomas. *Int J Radiat Oncol Biol Phys* 2002;52(2):514-21.

[37] Piva R, Cavalla P, Bortolotto S, Cordera S, Richiardi P, Schiffer D. *p27*/kip1 expression in human astrocytic gliomas. *Neurosci Lett* 1997;234(2-3):127-30.

[38] Morosetti R, Kawamata N, Gombart AF, Miller CW, Hatta Y, Hirama T, et al. Alterations of the *p27*KIP1 gene in non-Hodgkin's lymphomas and adult T-cell leukemia/lymphoma. *Blood* 1995;86(5):1924-30.

[39] Spirin KS, Simpson JF, Takeuchi S, Kawamata N, Miller CW, Koeffler HP. *p27*/Kip1 mutation found in breast cancer. *Cancer Res* 1996;56(10):2400-4.

[40] Farizan A, Asmarina K, Abdullah J, Jaafar H, Ghazali MM, Aini I, et al. Screening of Cyclin Dependent Kinase Inhibitor *p27* and Cyclin D1 gene in association with gliomas and meningiomas in Malaysia. *The Malaysian Journal of Medical Sciences* 2005;12:240.

[41] Shigemasa K, Tanimoto H, Parham GP, Parmley TH, Ohama K, O'Brien TJ. Cyclin D1 overexpression and p53 mutation status in epithelial ovarian cancer. *J Soc Gynecol Investig* 1999;6(2):102-8.

[42] Sundarrajan M, Gupta S, Rao KV. Overexpression of cyclin D1 is associated with the decondensation of chromatin during den-induced sequential hepatocarcinogenesis. *Cell Biol Int* 2002;26(8):699-706.

[43] Cordon-Cardo C. Mutations of cell cycle regulators. Biological and clinical implications for human neoplasia. *Am J Pathol* 1995;147(3):545-60.

[44] Koontongkaew S, Chareonkitkajorn L, Chanvitan A, Leelakriangsak M, Amornphimoltham P. Alterations of p53, pRb, cyclin D(1) and cdk4 in human oral and pharyngeal squamous cell carcinomas. *Oral Oncol* 2000;36(4):334-9.

[45] Rousseau A, Lim MS, Lin Z, Jordan RC. Frequent cyclin D1 gene amplification and protein overexpression in oral epithelial dysplasias. *Oral Oncol* 2001;37(3):268-75.

[46] Cheung TH, Yu MM, Lo KW, Yim SF, Chung TK, Wong YF. Alteration of cyclin D1 and CDK4 gene in carcinoma of uterine cervix. *Cancer Lett* 2001;166(2):199-206.

[47] Nishimoto IN, Pinheiro NA, Rogatto SR, Carvalho AL, Simpson AJ, Caballero OL, et al. Cyclin D1 gene polymorphism as a risk factor for squamous cell carcinoma of the upper aerodigestive system in non-alcoholics. *Oral Oncol* 2004;40(6):604-10.

[48] Kong S, Amos CI, Luthra R, Lynch PM, Levin B, Frazier ML. Effects of cyclin D1 polymorphism on age of onset of hereditary nonpolyposis colorectal cancer. *Cancer Res* 2000;60(2):249-52.

[49] Moreno-Bueno G, Rodriguez-Perales S, Sanchez-Estevez C, Hardisson D, Sarrio D, Prat J, et al. Cyclin D1 gene (CCND1) mutations in endometrial cancer. *Oncogene* 2003;22(38):6115-8.

[50] Liou AK, Clark RS, Henshall DC, Yin XM, Chen J. To die or not to die for neurons in ischemia, traumatic brain injury and epilepsy: a review on the stress-activated signaling pathways and apoptotic pathways. *Prog Neurobiol* 2003;69(2):103-42.

[51] Bast BT, Pogrel MA, Regezi JA. The expression of apoptotic proteins and matrix metalloproteinases in odontogenic myxomas. *J Oral Maxillofac Surg* 2003;61(12):1463-6.

[52] Evan GI, Vousden KH. Proliferation, cell cycle and apoptosis in cancer. *Nature* 2001;411(6835):342-8.

[53] Kuhlmann T, Glas M, zum Bruch C, Mueller W, Weber A, Zipp F, et al. Investigation of bax, bcl-2, bcl-x and p53 gene polymorphisms in multiple sclerosis. *J Neuroimmunol* 2002; 129(1-2):154-60.

[54] McGill G, Fisher DE. Apoptosis in tumorigenesis and cancer therapy. *Front Biosci* 1997; 2:d353-79.

[55] Rampino N, Yamamoto H, Ionov Y, Li Y, Sawai H, Reed JC, et al. Somatic frameshift mutations in the BAX gene in colon cancers of the microsatellite mutator phenotype. *Science* 1997; 275(5302):967-9.

[56] Sakuragi N, Salah-eldin AE, Watari H, Itoh T, Inoue S, Moriuchi T, et al. Bax, Bcl-2, and p53 expression in endometrial cancer. *Gynecol Oncol* 2002; 86(3):288-96.

[57] Asmarina K, Abdullah J, Jaafar H, Aini I, Manaf A. Alteration of Bax gene in brain tumors. *Journal of Clinical Neuroscience 2004;* 11(supplement 1):S103.

[58] Levicar N, Nuttall RK, Lah TT. Proteases in brain tumour progression. *Acta Neurochir* (Wien) 2003; 145(9):825-38.

[59] McCawley LJ, Matrisian LM. Matrix metalloproteinases: multifunctional contributors to tumor progression. *Mol Med Today* 2000; 6(4):149-56.

[60] Curran S, Murray GI. Matrix metalloproteinases: molecular aspects of their roles in tumour invasion and metastasis. *Eur J Cancer* 2000;36(13 Spec No):1621-30.

[61] Ghilardi G, Biondi ML, Mangoni J, Leviti S, DeMonti M, Guagnellini E, et al. Matrix metalloproteinase-1 promoter polymorphism 1G/2G is correlated with colorectal cancer invasiveness. *Clin Cancer Res* 2001; 7(8):2344-6.

[62] Fang S, Jin X, Wang R, Li Y, Guo W, Wang N, et al. Polymorphisms in the MMP1 and MMP3 promoter and non-small cell lung carcinoma in North China. *Carcinogenesis* 2005; 26(2):481-6.

[63] Ye S, Eriksson P, Hamsten A, Kurkinen M, Humphries SE, Henney AM. Progression of coronary atherosclerosis is associated with a common genetic variant of the human stromelysin-1 promoter which results in reduced gene expression. *J Biol Chem* 1996;271(22):13055-60.

[64] Ghilardi G, Biondi ML, Caputo M, Leviti S, DeMonti M, Guagnellini E, et al. A single nucleotide polymorphism in the matrix metalloproteinase-3 promoter enhances breast cancer susceptibility. *Clin Cancer Res* 2002;8(12):3820-3.

[65] Hirata H, Okayama N, Naito K, Inoue R, Yoshihiro S, Matsuyama H, et al. Association of a haplotype of matrix metalloproteinase (MMP)-1 and MMP-3 polymorphisms with renal cell carcinoma. *Carcinogenesis* 2004;25(12):2379-84.

[66] Smolarz B, Szyllo K, Romanowicz-Makowska H, Niewiadomski M, Kozlowska E, Kulig A. PCR analysis of matrix metalloproteinase 3 (MMP-3) gene promoter polymorphism in ovarian cancer. *Pol J Pathol* 2003;54(4):233-8.

[67] Asmarina K, Abdullah J, Farizan A, Jaafar H, Ghazali MM, Aini I, et al. Preliminary Report Of Genetic Variation In Human Stromelysin 1 Promoter In Gliomas And Meningiomas. In: *6th National Congress on Genetics;* 2005; Kuala Lumpur (Malaysia); 2005. p. 192-193.

[68] Gomori E, Doczi T, Pajor L, Matolcsy A. Sporadic p53 mutations and absence of ras mutations in glioblastomas. *Acta Neurochir* (Wien) 1999;141(6):593-9.

[69] Watzinger F, Lion T. RAS family. In: *Atlas of genetics and cytogenetics in oncology and haematology;* 1999.

[70] Isobe T, Hiyama K, Yoshida Y, Fujiwara Y, Yamakido M. Prognostic significance of p53 and ras gene abnormalities in lung adenocarcinoma patients with stage I disease after curative resection. *Jpn J Cancer Res* 1994;85(12):1240-6.

[71] Yusoff AA, J.Abdullah, H.Jaafar, Aini I, Manaf A, Khatijah Y, et al. The lack of a role for ras gene in human gliomas in Malaysian patients. *The Malaysian Journal of Medical Sciences,* 2004;11(1):145.

[72] Zan MSM, Fauzi ARM, Yusoff AA, Ghazali MM, Abdullah J, Aini I, et al. Molecular Studies of NF2 and Ras Family Gene in Malaysian Human Brain Tumors. *Med J Malaysia* 2003.;58 (Supplement E):102.

[73] Ghazali MM, Zan MSM, Fauzi ARM, Yusoff AA, Abdullah J, Aini I, et al. Ras, c-myc and epidermal growth factor receptor (EGFR) gene alteration in human gliomas in

North East Malaysian patients. *The Malaysian Journal of Medical Sciences*, 2005; 12(Suppl 1):161.

[74] SÜZEN S, PARRY JM. Analysis of ras Gene Mutation in Human Oral Tumours by Polymerase Chain Reaction and Direct Sequencing. *Tr. J. of Med. Sci.* 2001; 31:217-223.

[75] Halter SA, Webb L, Rose J. Lack of ras mutations and prediction of long-term survival in carcinoma of the colon. *Mod Pathol* 1992;5(2):131-4.

[76] Bishop JM. Retroviruses and cancer genes. *Adv.Cancer Res* 1982; 37:1-32.

[77] Sheiness D, L.Fanshier, Bishop JM. Identification of nucleotide sequences which may encode the oncogenic capacity of avian retrovirus MC29. *J.Virol* 1978; 28:600-610.

[78] Cole MD. The myc oncogene; its role in transformation and differentiation. *Annu.Rev.Genet.* 1986;20:361-384.

[79] Dalla-Favera, R EPG, S.Martinotti, G.Faranchini, T.S.Papas, Gallo RC, et al. Cloning and characterization of different human sequences related to the onc gene (v-myc) of avian myelocytomatosis virus (MC29). *Proc. Natl. Acad. Sci USA* 1982; 79: 6497-6501.

[80] Dang CV, L.A.Lee. c-myc function in neoplasia. R.G. *Landes and Springer-Verlag,* Austin, Tex. 1995.

[81] Facchini LM, Penn LZ. The molecular role of Myc in growth and transformation: recent discoveries lead to new insights. *Faseb J* 1998; 12(9):633-51.

[82] Peng H, Diss T, Isaacson PG, Pan L. c-myc gene abnormalities in mucosa-associated lymphoid tissue (MALT) lymphomas. *J Pathol* 1997; 181(4):381-6.

[83] Jain M, Arvanitis C, Chu K, Dewey W, Leonhardt E, Trinh M, et al. Sustained loss of a neoplastic phenotype by brief inactivation of MYC. *Science* 2002;297(5578):102-4.

[84] Peng H, Du M, Ji J, Isaacson PG, Pan L. High-resolution SSCP analysis using polyacrylamide agarose composite gel and a background-free silver staining method. *Biotechniques* 1995; 19(3):410-4.

[85] Blackwood EM, R.N.Eisenman. Myc and Max function as a nucleoprotein complex. *Curr. Opin. Genet. Dev.* 1991; 2:227-235.

[86] Mazira Mohamad Ghazali, Shahril Mohd Zan, Abdul Aziz Yusoff, Jafri Abdullah, Hasnan Jaafar, Abdul Rahman Arif et al. Absence of ras, c-myc and Epidermal Growth Factor Receptor (EGFR) mutation in human gliomas in the North East Malaysian patients and its clinical factors associated with pathological grading after 5 years of diagnosis. *Malaysian Journal of Medical Sciences.* 2005; 12 (2): 27-33

[87] Little CD, Nau MM, Carney DN, Gazdar AF, J.D.Minna. Amplification and expression of the c-myc oncogene in human lung cancer cell lines. *Nature* 1983; 306:194-196.

[88] Munzel P, D.Marx, H.Kochel, A.Schauer, K.W.Bock. Genomic alterations of the c-myc protooncogene in relation to the overexpression of c-erbB2 and Ki-67 in human breast and cervix carcinomas. *J Cancer Res. Clin. Oncol* 1991; 117: 603-607.

[89] Augenlicht LH, S.Wadler, G.Corner, C.Richards, L.Ryan, A.S.Multani, et al. Low-level c-myc amplification in human colonic carcinoma cell lines and tumors: a frequent, p53-independent mutation associated with improved outcome in a randomized multi-institutional trial. *Cancer Res.* 1997; 57:1769-1775.

[90] Malaysia Ministry of Health. Annual report. 1999.

[91] Kanzawa T, Ito H, Kondo Y, Kondo S. Current and Future Gene Therapy for Malignant Gliomas. *J Biomed Biotechnol* 2003; 1:25-34.

[92] Abdul Rahman Omar, Aini Ideris, Abdul Manaf Ali, Fauziah Othman, Khatijah Yusoff, Jafri Malin Abdullah, Haryati Shila Mohamad Wali, Madihah Zawawi and Narayani Meyyappan. An overview on the development of Newcastle disease virus as an anti-cancer therapy. *Malaysian Journal of Medical Sciences.* 2003; 10: 4-12

[93] Mohd Azmi Mohd Lila, John Shia Kwong Siew, Hayati Zakaria, Suria Mohd Saad, Lim Shen Ni and Jafri Malin Abdullah. Cell Targeting in Anti-Cancer Gene Therapy. *Malaysian Journal of Medical Sciences.* 2004; 11: 9-23

In: Focus on Brain Cancer Research
Editor: Andrew V. Yang, pp. 99-111
ISBN 1-59454-973-7

Chapter VI

Histopathological Analysis on Proliferative Potentials of Recurrent and Non-Recurrent Meningiomas

Akira Matsuno[1*], Takamitsu Fujimaki[2], Tadashi Nagashima[1], Takaaki Kirino[3] and R. Yoshiyuki Osamura[4]

[1] Department of Neurosurgery, Teikyo University Ichihara Hospital, Chiba, Japan
[2] Department of Neurosurgery, Teikyo University Itabashi Hospital, Tokyo, Japan
[3] Department of Neurosurgery, University of Tokyo Hospital, Tokyo, Japan
[4] Department of Pathology, Tokai University School of Medicine, Kanagawa, Japan

Abstract

Proliferative potentials of 127 patients with meningioma were examined according to an immunohistochemical staining method using an anti-Ki-67 monoclonal antibody, MIB-1, for paraffin sections, and the correlations among MIB-1 staining index (SI), histopathological finding, and clinical course of the disease were analyzed retrospectively. The mean MIB-1 SI of 50 male patients with meningioma was 5.5%, whereas that of 77 female patients was 2.7%. High MIB-1 SI was observed in younger patients. These age- and sex-related differences in MIB-1 SI were statistically significant. All the patients were divided into 3 groups: 73 patients with non-recurrent meningioma; 21 patients with recurrent meningioma in whom the specimens obtained during the initial surgery were used to calculate the MIB-1 SI; 33 patients with recurrent meningioma in whom the specimens obtained during the surgery for recurrent tumors were used to calculate the MIB-1 SI. The mean MIB-1 staining indices in these patients were 1.6%, 3.6%, and 8.8%, respectively, and there were statistically significant differences among

* Correspondence: Akira Matsuno, M.D., Ph.D. Department of Neurosurgery, Teikyo University Ichihara Hospital, 3426-3 Anesaki, Ichihara City, Chiba 299-0111, Japan; Tel: 81-436-62-1211; Fax: 81-436-62-1357

these three groups. Statistical analyses revealed that meningiomas with MIB-1 SI of 3% or higher have significantly high tendency for recurrence in clinical courses, especially in the first 10 year-follow-up periods. Moreover, there is statistically significant correlation between MIB-1 SI and recurrence in each Simpson's grade. Time interval to the next recurrence in recurrent meningiomas is associated with proliferative potential as demonstrated by MIB-1 SI, and a formula of correlation has been proposed to predict the date of the next recurrence. The examination on proliferative potentials of meningiomas using MIB-1 SI is very important for biological and histopathological analyses and the prediction of future recurrence. The mean BrdU labelling index (LI) of recurrent meningiomas was reported to be significantly higher than that of the non-recurrent meningiomas. BrdU LI also can predict the time to re-operation. BrdU LI, MIB-1 SI, and tumor doubling time of intracranial meningiomas have mutual relationship. Many other biological or genetic variables can affect the proliferation of tumors, and nevertheless, BrdU LI and MIB-1 SI are closely related to clinical recurrence or regrowth of meningiomas.

Key Words: meningioma, MIB-1, Ki-67, BrdU, proliferative potential, recurrence

Introduction

Meningiomas are common, usually benign, tumors of the meninges arising from the arachnoid cells. They are a heterogeneous group of tumors that are categorized into 15 subtypes [27]. Several investigators have studied the clinical and biological features of recurrent and non-recurrent meningiomas [3, 8, 10, 11, 14, 20, 21, 31, 37, 38, 54]. Moreover, in recent years, meningiomas have been analyzed by histopathological examination focused on proliferative potentials. Representative studies on proliferative potentials include bromodeoxyuridine (BrdU) labeling index (LI) [16, 22, 53], proliferative cell nuclear antigen (PCNA) [24], argyrophilic nucleolar organizer region (AgNOR) count [4, 9, 45], and Ki-67 or MIB-1 staining index (SI) [1, 2, 15, 18, 22, 23, 26, 28-30, 32, 33, 35, 36, 39, 42, 44, 45, 48-51, 56, 57]. In this chapter, proliferative potentials of intracranial meningiomas, represented by Ki-67 SI, were focused, and their correlations with histopathological findings, recurrence and tumor growth were discussed with review on literature.

Materials and Methods

We examined proliferative potentials of 127 intracranial meningiomas by MIB-1 immunohistochemical staining method for paraffin sections. They comprised 50 males and 77 females, with the mean age of 50.9 years. There were 54 patients with recurrent meningioma (42.5%). The correlations among MIB-1 SI, histopathological finding, and clinical course of the disease were analyzed retrospectively [32].

The details of MIB-1 immunohistochemical staining method were described in our previous report [32], and in this chapter the method was shown briefly as follows. Four μm sections of the routinely processed paraffin blocks were deparaffinized in xylene, and rehydrated through graded ethanol to water. Following blockage of the endogenous peroxidase activity with 0.3% H2O2 in methanol for 30 minutes, the slides were dipped in 0.01 M citrate pH 6.0, and the Ki-67 antigen was retrieved with microwave irradiation for 30 minutes (10 times for 3 minutes). They were immunostained with a commercially available anti-Ki-67 monoclonal antibody, MIB-1 (mouse, diluted 1:100 in bovine serum albumin (BSA) - phosphate buffered saline pH 7.4 (PBS)) (Immunotech S.A., Marseille, France), at room temperature for 1 hour. The biotinylated antibody against mouse immunoglobulin (IgG) (goat, Vectastain; Vector Laboratories Inc., Burlingame, Ca., USA) was applied as a secondary antibody for 30 minutes. Immunoreactions were followed by streptavidin and biotin complex (ABC) labeled with horseradish peroxidase using Vectastain's ABC kit (Vector Laboratories Inc., Burlingame, Ca., USA) for 30 minutes, and developed with freshly prepared 3,3'-diaminobendizine tetrahydrochloride dissolved in 0.05 M Tris-HCl pH 7.6 and 0.017% H2O2 for 7 minutes. Nuclear staining was carried out with hematoxylin for 5 seconds. The entire tissue sections were examined under high power magnification (x400). The number of cells stained positively with MIB-1 and the total number of tumor cells were counted in several representative fields containing more than 1,000 cells in total. Their ratio was indicated as MIB-1 SI (%). In the areas of heterogeneous distribution of MIB-1 immunopositive cells, the area containing the largest number of MIB-1 immunostained cells was regarded as the area representing the proliferative activity of the tumor. The mean MIB-1 SI and its standard deviation (SD) of each corresponding group were calculated and their correlation was analyzed with Student's t-test.

Results

MIB-1 SI and Distribution of Age and Sex

The mean MIB-1 SI of 50 male patients with meningiomas was 5.5% (SD: 7.5), whereas that of 77 female patients was 2.7% (SD: 3.8). This sex-related difference in MIB-1 SI was statistically significant (P=0.003). High MIB-1 staining indices were observed in younger patients. For example, the mean MIB-1 SI of patients below age 40 was 7.4% (SD: 9.8), whereas that of patients aged 40 or over was 2.9% (SD: 3.4). This age-related difference in MIB-1 SI was also statistically significant (P=0.0001).

MIB-1 SI and Location of Meningioma

Our series comprised patients with the following subtypes of meningioma: 32 convexity, 15 parasagittal, 3 falx, 20 sphenoid ridge, 8 tentorial, 15 tuberculum sellae or olfactory groove and 5 intraventricular meningiomas [32]. Twenty-five patients with skull base meningiomas, such as those located in cerebellopontine angle, petroclival or cavernous sinus regions, as well as 4 patients with meningiomas located in the other regions, were also included in our series. Their mean MIB-1 staining indices were 5.5% (SD: 8.5), 3.6 % (SD:

2.0), 1.2% (SD: 0.4), 3.2% (SD: 3.0), 1.9% (SD: 1.3), 2.1% (SD: 3.4), 6.7% (SD: 4.6), 4.1% (SD: 6.7), and 2.3% (SD: 2.1), respectively. There was no statistically significant relationship between tumor location and MIB-1 SI (P-values were higher than 0.05 in all comparisons between MIB-1 SI and tumor location).

MIB-1 SI and Histopathological Subtypes of Meningiomas

We found that there was statistical significant difference in the averages of MIB-1 SI between atypical meningioma (6.1%) and meningotheliomatous (2.1%), or fibroblastic meningioma (3.0%) [32]. Anaplastic (malignant) meningioma was found to have an extremely high mean MIB-1 SI (26.5%,) compared with that of other subtypes of meningiomas [32].

MIB-1 SI and Recurrence or Regrowth of Meningiomas

We divided all the patients into 3 groups: 73 patients with non-recurrent meningioma; 21 patients with recurrent meningioma in whom the specimens obtained during the initial surgery were used to calculate the MIB-1 SI; 33 patients with recurrent meningioma in whom the specimens obtained during the surgery for recurrent tumors were used to calculate the MIB-1 SI. The mean MIB-1 staining indices of non-recurrent tumors, recurrent tumors at the first operation, and recurrent tumors at the re-operation were 1.6%, 3.6%, and 8.8%, respectively, and that there were statistically significant differences among these three groups [32].

MIB-1 SI and Recurrence or Regrowth of Meningiomas in Relation to the Extent of Tumor Removal

Some reports have shown that the degree of surgical removal, namely, Simpson's grading, is closely related to future recurrence [3, 8, 11, 27, 29]. Then, in order to predict the future recurrence of meningioma on the basis of MIB-1 SI of meningiomas more precisely, the tumors should be assigned to each group of Simpson's grade and the relationship between MIB-1 SI and recurrence should be analyzed individually. There was a statistically significant correlation between recurrence and MIB-1 SI in meningiomas that were assigned to each Simpson's grade according to the extent of tumor removal [32].

Time Interval to the Next Recurrence and MIB-1 SI

Time interval to the next recurrence in recurrent meningiomas was associated with proliferative potential as demonstrated by MIB-1 SI, and a formula of correlation was proposed to predict the date of the next recurrence [32].

Y=125.82-96.447xLog(X)
X=MIB-1 SI (%)
Y=Time interval to the next recurrence (months)

Cut-off Point of MIB-1 SI that Can Predict Recurrence or Regrowth

Kaplan-Meyer analysis elucidated that meningiomas with MIB-1 SI of 3% or higher had significantly high tendency for recurrence in clinical courses, especially in the first 10 year-follow-up periods [32].

Discussion

MiB-1 Immunohistochemistry in Meningioma

Immunohistochemical staining of the Ki-67 antigen is capable of detecting all proliferative cells [7, 13, 22, 25, 29, 32-34, 44, 46]. An anti-Ki-67 monoclonal antibody, MIB-1, has become available for the analysis of proliferative potentials of tumors using the routinely processed paraffin sections.

We found that there was statistical significant difference in the averages of MIB-1 SI between atypical meningioma (6.1%) and meningotheliomatous (2.1%), or fibroblastic meningioma (3.0%) [32]. Malignant (anaplastic) meningioma had an extremely high mean MIB-1 SI (26.5%,) [32]. Other several reports conducted that the mean MIB-1 SI for benign meningiomas ranged from 0.7 to 2.2%, that for atypical meningiomas ranged from 2.1 to 9.3%, and that for anaplastic meningiomas ranged from 11.0 to 16.3% [1, 26, 28, 45]. Perry et al. described that MIB-1 SI appeared to be of greatest value in the evaluation of tumors exhibiting borderline atypia [49]. These studies demonstrated that MIB-1 SI was mostly in accordance with the histopathological grading of meningioma.

In our study, the mean MIB-1 SIs of non-recurrent tumors, recurrent tumors at the first operation, and recurrent tumors at the re-operation were 1.6%, 3.6%, and 8.8%, respectively, and that there were statistically significant differences among these three groups [32]. Other reports demonstrated that the mean MIB-1 SI of non-recurrent meningiomas ranged from 0.98 to 3.8 %, whereas that of recurrent meningiomas ranged from 4.0 to 8.8 % [1, 28, 32, 46]. Recent report by Roser et al. also found that MIB-1 SI is significantly correlated with WHO grading of meningioma [51]. These studies showed the significant correlation of MIB-1 SI with recurrence of meningioma.

We demonstrated that there is a statistically significant correlation between recurrence and MIB-1 SI in meningiomas that were assigned to each Simpson's grade according to the extent of tumor removal [32]. Roser et al. found that MIB-1 SI was independent of the resection grade, Simpson's grading (grade1; 5.75%, 2; 4.2%, 3; 6.76%, and 4; 7.99%) [51]. It may be true that the extent of surgical removal is related to future recurrence, however, in each grading of surgical removal, MIB-1 SI that has relationship with histopathological grading is closely related to future recurrence or regrowth of meningiomas.

Time interval to the next recurrence in recurrent meningiomas is associated with proliferative potential as demonstrated by MIB-1 SI. We can predict the time interval to the next recurrence using the above stated formula. This formula can predict the period of the recurrence of meningiomas with a high proliferative potential represented by MIB-1 SI.

We have shown, by Kaplan-Meyer method, that meningiomas with MIB-1 SI of 3% or higher have significantly high tendency for recurrence in clinical courses, especially in the first 10 year-follow-up periods [32]. The other cut-off points predicting recurrence identified in the previous reports were 3.0% [18], 3.2% [45], 4.0% [51], 4.2% [49], and 10% [15].

We should note that there are some variations among researches of MIB-1 SI of meningiomas. These variations may be due to the differences in staining and counting methodologies among different laboratories. Usually antigen retrieval of Ki-67 is carried out in MIB-1 immunohistochemistry. Munakata et al. stated that microwave oven heating for at least 14 min yielded significant antigen retrieval of Ki-67 in MIB-1 immunohistochemistry using routinely processed paraffin sections [40]. Recent researchers have carried out sufficient antigen retrieval in MIB-1 immunohistochemistry. Therefore, the counting methodology that may differ among researchers is the main reason for the variations of MIB-1 SI of meningiomas among researchers. Nakasu et al. evaluated the predictability of MIB-1 immunohistochemistry for growth and recurrences of meningiomas using two different counting methods: 1) in the area of the highest MIB-1 staining (HL method) and 2) in randomly selected fields (RS method). The MIB-1 SI determined by the HL method was approximately twice as high as that by the RS method [45]. Thus, in order to predict the future recurrence or regrowth of meningiomas more precisely, researchers should analyze their own materials and use their standard cut-off points in their own laboratories.

There are some reports suggesting that MIB-1 SI is not correlated with tumor behavior [1, 39, 51]. Abramovich and Prayson [1] reported the absence of a significant difference in MIB-1 SI between 32 recurrent and 27 non-recurrent meningiomas. Møller and Brœndstrup [39] also found negative difference in MIB-1 SI between 26 recurrent and 17 non-recurrent meningiomas. They found that PCNA was also of minor value as predictors of recurrence of benign meningiomas. The materials these authors analyzed comprised a relatively small number of tumors. Roser et al. stated that MIB-1 SI was not a statistically significant predictor of survival time in totally excised WHO grade I meningiomas [51]. Their analyses excluded WHO grade 2 and 3 meningiomas and subtotally or partially resected meningiomas. Meanwhile, they proposed that the cut-off point of MIB-1 SI for prediction of future recurrence is 4%. In summary, those reports that found negative correlation between MIB-1 SI and recurrence of meningiomas belong to a minor group. As stated above, most of the reports showed the significant correlation of MIB-1 SI with clinical outcome.

Some authors stated that other factors are also important to predict the future recurrence. Hsu et al. analyzed the expression of transforming growth factor (TGF) ▪ ▪ and MIB-1 SI in 57 intracranial meningiomas [18]. They found that the overexpression of TGF ▪ is associated with tumor progression, and that it is, as well as MIB-1 SI, an important prognostic indicator for patients with meningiomas. Yamasaki et al. suggested that high levels of vascular endothelial growth factor (VEGF) expression are significantly related to the recurrence of meningioma, and that VEGF secretion from microscopic residue remaining after surgery may induce neovascularization, which promotes the recurrence of meningioma

[57]. As to the p53 immunohistochemistry, we found the close relationship among p53 immunoreactivity, MIB-1 SI, and recurrence [33]. Karamitopoulou et al. found that a good correlation exists between histological grading, MIB-1 and p53 protein expression in meningiomas [26]. Nagashima et al. stated that accumulation of p53 protein associated with highly proliferative potentials is a common and characteristic feature that may indicate malignant biological behavior in meningiomas. In contrast, Perry et al. suggested that, regarding patients with primary gross totally resected meningiomas, neither flow cytometry nor p53 immunohistochemistry provides useful prognostic information [49]. Karamitopoulou et al. found that the presence of bcl-2 protein expression, together with high MIB-1 SI, is associated with unfavorable prognosis of the benign meningiomas [26]. Wolfsberger et al. stated that low expression of progesterone receptor is related with the histological grade of meningiomas and MIB-1 SI [56]. Roser et al. found a significant correlation between negative progesteron-receptor status and high tumor vascularity with high MIB-1 SI [51]. The significant correlation of high vascularity and high MIB-1 SI suggests the neoangiogenetic capacity of meningiomas [5, 19]. High progesterone receptor status in benign meningiomas is reported to be associated with lower recurrence rate and vice versa [6, 12].

MIB-1 SI has been applied to clinical and histopathological studies of other malignant tumors such as a gastric cancer [41, 52]. Setala et al. indicated that p53 protein expression may be of prognostic significance in gastric cancer, while PCNA and Ki-67 antigen expression have no predictive value [52]. Meanwhile, Nagazato et al. stated that the maximum tumor diameter, mitotic index, and Ki-67 antigen expression are useful as an index of malignancy for gastric stromal tumor [41]. Such malignant tumors have more genetic or biological abnormalities than meningiomas, and thus the relevance of MIB-1 SI with clinical outcome may be less important.

To summarize the evaluation of MIB-1 SI in meningiomas in the literature, most reports conducted the significant relationship between MIB-1 SI and clinical outcome, although other biological or genetic variables may affect the proliferation of tumors [15, 18, 22, 23, 26, 28-30, 32, 33, 35, 36, 44, 45, 48-50, 56, 57]. Therefore, the examination on proliferative potentials of meningiomas using MIB-1 SI is very important for biological and histopathological analyses and the prediction of future recurrence.

Tumor Volume Doubling Time (Td) and Ki-67

Nakaguchi et al. [44] clarified that MIB-1 immunohistochemical study is useful for determining the rate of regrowth for postoperative residual tumors. They measured tumor volume of 29 intracranial meningiomas from 22 patients by using digital planimeter and computed tomography or magnetic resonance imaging neuroimages. Td was determined by the following formula.

$$Td = t \times \log 2 / (\log Vb - \mathrm{Log}\ Va)$$

Va: initial tumor volume

Vb: tumor volume at t days after Va

There was a strong inverse correlation between log(Td) and MIB-1 SI ($P < 0.001$).

Log Td = 31.4 – 0.14 x MIB-1 SI

Based on this formula, we can predict the regrowth potential of a meningioma after initial surgery.

BrdU LI and Recurrence

BrdU can detect S phase cells alone [16, 53, 55], and histopathological studies using BrdU LI require intravenous injection of BrdU prior to surgery, or incubation of cultured tumor cells with BrdU. The method of BrdU immunohistochemical stainings was described in several reports [16, 17, 22, 43, 53].

Hoshino et al. analyzed BrdU LIs of 20 intracranial meningiomas [16]. In their report, the average LIs for non-malignant (11 cases) and histologically malignant meningiomas (7 cases) were 0.45% and 3.9% respectively ($P<0.05$). Nine of 20 meningiomas had a LI greater than 1%, and 6 of those 9 (67%) were recurrent. They concluded that meningiomas with a LI greater than 1% appeared to grow faster and recurred more frequently than those with LIs less than 1%. They suggested that the higher LI might indicate biological malignancy.

Shibuya et al. reported that 53 of 178 meningiomas had BrdU LIs greater than or equal to 1% [53]. Of these 53 tumors, 21 were diagnosed histopathologically as malignant meningioma. The mean BrdU LI of recurrent tumors (mean±SD: 3.9±2.6 %) was significantly higher than that of the non-recurrent tumors (1.9±1.0%) ($P<0.005$). They showed, by logarithmic regression analysis, that BrdU LI could predict the time to re-operation.

Y=70.0 x X-1.2 (R = 0.76)
X=BrdU LI (%)
Y=Time interval to the re-operation (months)

This formula can be used to predict the period of the recurrence of meningiomas with a high proliferative potential represented by BrdU LI.

Kakinuma et al. [22] reported that the average of BUdR LI for non-recurrent meningiomas was 0.77±0.13% (mean±SD), and that recurrent meningiomas had significantly higher LI at the first operation (3.77±1.22%). The recurrent ratio significantly increased with the degree of BUdR LI.

Thus, the BrdU LI study is useful for the analyses of proliferative potentials and biological behaviors of meningiomas. However, the BrdU LI study is inappropriate for retrospective studies, since it requires intravenous injection of BrdU prior to surgery or incubation of cultured tumor cells with BrdU. Then, MIB-1 immunohistochemistry has much wider applicability to histopathological studies of tumors, and thus, in this review article, MIB-1 immunohistochemistry is described more extensively as follows.

BrdU LI and MIB-1 SI

Kakinuma et al. examined the reciprocal relationship among BrdU LI, MIB-1 SI, and Td of recurrent meningiomas [22]. In their series of 182 primary intracranial meningiomas, 46 cases recurred. The averages of BrdU LI and MIB-1 SI for non-recurrent meningiomas were $0.77 \pm 0.13\%$ (mean$\pm$SD) and $4.71 \pm 1.96\%$, respectively. Meanwhile, the averages of BrdU LI and MIB-1 SI for recurrent meningiomas at the first operation were $3.77 \pm 1.22\%$ and $14.78 \pm 3.17\%$, respectively. Their linear regression analysis demonstrated a significant correlation between BrdU LI and MIB-1 SI.

$$\text{BrdU LI} = 0.234 + 0.98 \times \text{MIB-1 SI}$$

They also calculated accurately, by NIH computer software, Td, which showed a significant inverse correlation with each of the indices.

$$\text{Td} = -409.609 \times \log \text{BrdU LI} + 368.258$$
$$\text{Td} = -416.008 \times \log \text{MIB-1 SI} + 730.704$$

They concluded that BrdU LI, MIB-1 SI and Td of individual tumors correlate mutually well.

Langford et al. [29] analyzed proliferative potentials of meningiomas from 40 adult patients immunohistochemically using BrdU LI and MIB-1 SI. They also found a good correlation between the BrdU and MIB-1 proliferation markers.

Thus, BrdU LI, MIB-1 SI and Td of intracranial meningiomas are considered to have mutual correlation.

Conclusion

Both BrdU and MIB-1 immunohistochemistry are useful for proliferative potentials of intracranial meningiomas. Many other biological or genetic variables may affect the proliferation of tumors, and nevertheless, BrdU LI and MIB-1 SI are closely related with clinical recurrence or regrowth of meningiomas.

References

[1] Abramovich, C.M. and Prayson, R.A. (1998) MIB-1 labeling indices in benign, aggressive, and malignant meningiomas: a study of 90 tumors. *Hum. Pathol.* 29:1420-1427.

[2] Abramovich, C.M. and Prayson, R.A. (1999) Histopathologic features and MIB-1 labeling indices in recurrent and nonrecurrent meningiomas. *Arch. Pathol. Lab. Med.* 123:793-800.

[3] Adegbite, A.B., Khan, M.I., Paine, K.W.E. and Tan, L.K. (1983) The recurrence of intracranial meningiomas after surgical treatment. *J. Neurosurg.* 58; 51-56.

[4] Bagni, A., Botticelli, A., Martinelli, A., Azzoni, P. and Trentini, G.P. (1991) AgNOR counts in recurrent and non-recurrent meningiomas. *Histopathology* 19; 465-467.

[5] Bitzer, M., Opitz, H., Popp, J., Morgalla, M., Gruber, A., Heiss, E. and Voigt, K. (1998) Angiogenesis and brain oedema in intracranial meningiomas: influence of vascular endothelial growth factor. *Acta Neurochir* (Wien). 140:333-340.

[6] Brandis, A., Mirzai, S., Tatagiba, M., Walter, G.F., Samii, M. and Ostertag, H. (1993) Immunohistochemical detection of female sex hormone receptors in meningiomas: correlation with clinical and histological features. *Neurosurgery* 33:212-217.

[7] Cattoretti, G., Becker, M.H.G., Key, G., Duchrow, M., Schlter, C., Galle, J. and Gerdes, J. (1992) Monoclonal antibodies against recombinant parts of the Ki-67 antigen (MIB1 and MIB3) detect proliferating cells in microwave-processed formalin-fixed paraffin sections. *J. Pathol.* 168; 357-363.

[8] Chan, R.C. and Thompson, G.B. (1984) Morbidity, mortality and quality of life following surgery for intracranial meningiomas. *J. Neurosurg.* 60; 52-60.

[9] Chin, L.S. and Hinton, D.R. (1991) The standardized assessment of argyrophilic nucleolar organizer regions in meningiomas. *J. Neurosurg.* 74; 590-596.

[10] Christensen, D., Laursen, H. and Klinken, L. (1983) Prediction of recurrence of meningiomas after surgical treatment: A quantitative approach. *Acta Neuropathol.* 61; 130-134.

[11] Crompton, M.R. and Gautier-Smith, P.C. (1970) The prediction of recurrence in meningiomas. *J. Neurol. Neurosurg. Psychiatry* 33; 80-87.

[12] Fewings, P.E., Battersby, R.D. and Timperley, W.R. (2000) Long-term follow up of progesterone receptor status in benign meningioma: a prognostic indicator of recurrence? *J. Neurosurg.* 92:401-405.

[13] Gerdes, J., Lemke, H., Baisch, H., Wacker, H.H., Schwab, U. and Stein, H. (1984) Cell cycle analysis of a cell proliferation-associated human nuclear antigen defined by the monoclonal antibody Ki-67. *J. Immunol.* 133; 1710-1715.

[14] Gupta, P.K., Sastry Kolluri, V.R., Das, S., Chandra Mouli, B.A., Narayana Swamy, K.S. and Dan, B.S. (1989) Recurrences in meningiomas after surgery. *Acta Neurochir* (Wien). 100; 104-109.

[15] Ho, D.M., Hsu, C.Y., Ting, L.T. and Chiang, H. (2002) Histopathology and MIB-1 labeling index predicted recurrence of meningiomas: a proposal of diagnostic criteria for patients with atypical meningioma. *Cancer* 94:1538-1547.

[16] Hoshino, T., Nagashima, T., Murovic, J.A., Wilson, C.B. and Davis, R.L. (1986) Proliferative potential of human meningiomas of brain. *Cancer* 58; 1466-1472.

[17] Hoshino, T., Nagashima, T., Cho, K.G., Davis, R.L., Donegan, J., Slusarz, M. and Wilson, C.B. (1989) Variability in the proliferative potential of human gliomas. *J. Neurooncol.* 7; 137-143.

[18] Hsu, D.W., Efird, J.T. and Hedley-Whyte, E.T. (1998) MIB-1 (Ki-67) index and transforming growth factor-alpha (TGF alpha) immunoreactivity are significant prognostic predictors for meningiomas. *Neuropathol. Appl. Neurobiol.* 24:441-452.

[19] Izycka-Swieszewska, E., Rzepko, R., Borowska-Lehman, J., Baranowska, E. and Warzocha, D. (1999) Recurrent meningiomas--the immunohistochemical analysis of angiogenesis and cellular proliferation. Preliminary study. *Folia Neuropathol.* 37:179-184.

[20] Jaaskelainen, J., Haltia, M. and Servo, A. (1986) Atypical and anaplastic meningiomas: Radiology, surgery, radiotherapy, and outcome. *Surg. Neurol.* 25; 233-242.

[21] Jellinger, K. and Slowik, F. (1975) Histological subtypes and prognostic problems in meningiomas. *J. Neurol.* 208; 279-298.

[22] Kakinuma, K., Tanaka, R., Onda, K. and Takahashi, H. (1998) Proliferative potential of recurrent intracranial meningiomas as evaluated by labelling indices of BUdR and Ki-67, and tumour doubling time. *Acta Neurochir* (Wien). 140; 26-31, discussion 31-32.

[23] Kalala, J.P., Benoit, D. and De Ridder, L. (2004) Can recurrence of meningiomas be predicted? *Anticancer Res.* 24:2319-2324.

[24] Karamitopoulou, E., Perentes, E., Melachrinou, M. and Maraziotis, T. (1993) Proliferating cell nuclear antigen immunoreactivity in human central nervous system neoplasms. *Acta Neuropathol.* 85; 316-322.

[25] Karamitopoulou, E., Perentes, E., Diamantis, I. and Maraziotis, T. (1994) Ki-67 immunoreactivity in human central nervous system neoplasms: a study with MIB1 monoclonal antibody on archival material. *Acta Neuropathol.* 87; 47-54.

[26] Karamitopoulou, E., Perentes, E., Tolnay, M. and Probst, A. (1998) Prognostic significance of MIB-1, p53, and bcl-2 immunoreactivity in meningiomas. *Hum. Pathol.* 29:140-145.

[27] Kleihues, P. and Cavenee, W.K. (2000) WHO classification of tumours of the nervous system. In *"Pathology and Genetics of Tumours of the Nervous System"*, ed. by P. Kleihues and W.K.,Cavenee, IARC Press, International Agency for Research on Cancer, Lyon, pp 6-7.

[28] Kolles, H., Niedermayer, I., Schmitt, C., Henn, W., Feld, R., Steudel, W.I., Zang, K.D. and Feiden, W. (1995) Triple approach for diagnosis and grading of meningiomas: histology, morphometry of Ki-67/Feulgen stainings, and cytogenetics. *Acta Neurochir* (Wien). 137:174-181.

[29] Langford, L.A., Cooksley, C.S. and DeMonte, F. (1996) Comparison of MIB-1 (Ki-67) antigen and bromodeoxyuridine proliferation indices in meningiomas. *Hum. Pathol.* 27; 350-354.

[30] Madsen, C. and Schroder, H.D. (1997) Ki-67 immunoreactivity in meningiomas--determination of the proliferative potential of meningiomas using the monoclonal antibody Ki-67. *Clin. Neuropathol.* 16:137-142.

[31] Marks, S.M., Whitwell, M.B. and Richard, H.L. (1986) Recurrence of meningiomas after operation. *Surg. Neurol.* 25; 436-440.

[32] Matsuno, A., Fujimaki, T., Sasaki, T., Nagashima, T., Ide, T., Asai, A,, Matsuura, R., Utsunomiya, H. and Kirino, T. (1996) Clinical and histopathological analysis of proliferative potentials of recurrent and non-recurrent meningiomas. *Acta Neuropathol.* 91; 504-510.

[33] Matsuno, A., Nagashima, T., Matsuura, R., Tanaka, H., Hirakawa, M., Murakami, M., Tamura, A. and Kirino, T. (1996) Correlation between MIB-1 staining index and the immunoreactivity of p53 protein in recurrent and non-recurrent meningiomas *Am. J. Clin. Pathol.* 106; 776-781.

[34] Matsuno, A., Sasaki, T., Nagashima, T., Kirino, T. and Osamura, R.Y. (2001) Proliferative potentials of intracranial chordomas with a reference to extracranial chordoma. *Acta Histochem. Cytochem.* 34; 305-312.

[35] Matsuno, A., Nakaguchi, H., Fujimaki, T. and Nagashima, T. (2005) Pathological and clinical analyses of proliferative potentials of meningiomas using MIB-1 staining index and tumor doubling time. *Recent Res. Devel. Human Pathol,* 2;1-8

[36] Matsuno, A., Nakaguchi, H., Nagashima, T., Fujimaki, T. and Osamura, R.Y. (2005) Histopathological analyses of proliferative potentials of intracranial meningiomas using bromodeoxyuridine and MIB-1 immunohistochemistry. *Acta Histochem Cytochem,* 38:9-15

[37] Melamed, S., Sahar, A. and Beller, A.J. (1979) The recurrence of intracranial meningioma. *Neurochirurgia* 22; 47-51.

[38] Mirimanoff, R.O., Dosoretz, D.E., Linggood, R.M., Ojemann, R.G. and Martuza, R.L. (1985) Meningioma: Analysis of recurrence and progression following neurosurgical resection. *J. Neurosurg.* 62; 18-24.

[39] Møller, M.L. and Brœndstrup, O. (1997) No prediction of recurrence of meningiomas by PCNA and Ki-67 immunohistochemistry. *J. Neurooncol.* 34:241-246.

[40] Munakata, S. and Hendricks, J.B. (1993) Effect of fixation time and microwave oven heating time on retrieval of the Ki-67 antigen from paraffin-embedded tissue. *J. Histochem. Cytochem.* 41:1241-1246.

[41] Nagasako, Y., Misawa, K., Kohashi, S., Hasegawa, K., Okawa, Y., Sano, H., Takada, A. and Sato, H. (2003) Evaluation of malignancy using Ki-67 labeling index for gastric stromal tumor. *Gastric Cancer* 6:168-172.

[42] Nagashima, G., Aoyagi, M., Yamamoto, M., Yamamoto, S., Wakimoto, H., Ohno, K., Yamamoto, K. and Hirakawa, K. (1999) P53 overexpression and proliferative potential in malignant meningiomas. *Acta Neurochir* (Wien). 141:53-61.

[43] Nagashima, T., Hoshino, T., Cho, K.G., Edwards, M.S., Hudgins, R.J. and Davis, R.L. (1988) The proliferative potential of human ependymomas measured by in situ bromodeoxyuridine labeling. *Cancer* 61; 2433-2438.

[44] Nakaguchi, H., Fujimaki, T., Matsuno, A., Matsuura, R., Asai, A., Suzuki, I., Sasaki, T. and Kirino, T. (1999) Postoperative residual tumor growth of meningioma can be predicted by MIB-1 immunohistochemistry. *Cancer* 85; 2249-2254.

[45] Nakasu, S., Li, D.H., Okabe, H., Nakajima, M. and Matsuda, M. (2001) Significance of MIB-1 staining indices in meningiomas: comparison of two counting methods. *Am. J. Surg. Pathol.* 25:472-478.

[46] Ohta, M., Iwaki, T., Kitamoto, T., Takeshita, I., Tateishi, J. and Fukui, M. (1994) MIB1 staining index and scoring of histologic features in meningiomas: Indicators for the prediction of biologic potential and proliferative management. *Cancer* 74; 3176-3189.

[47] Orita, T., Kajiwara, K., Nishizaki, T., Ikeda, N., Kamiryo, T. and Aoki, H. (1990) Nucleolar organizer regions in meningioma. *Neurosurgery* 26; 43-46.

[48] Paulus, W., Meixensberger, J., Hofmann, E. and Roggendorf, W. (1993) Effect of embolisation of meningioma on Ki-67 proliferation index. *J. Clin. Pathol.* 46; 876-877.

[49] Perry, A., Stafford, S.L., Scheithauer, B.W., Suman, V.J. and Lohse, C.M. (1998) The prognostic significance of MIB-1, p53, and DNA flow cytometry in completely resected primary meningiomas. *Cancer* 82:2262-2269.

[50] Prayson, R.A. (1996) Malignant meningioma: a clinicopathologic study of 23 patients including MIB1 and p53 immunohistochemistry. *Am. J. Clin. Pathol.* 105:719-726.

[51] Roser, F., Samii, M., Ostertag, H. and Bellinzona, M. (2004) The Ki-67 proliferation antigen in meningiomas. Experience in 600 cases. *Acta Neurochir* (Wien). 146:37-44.

[52] Setala, L., Kosma, V.M., Lipponen, P., Naukkarinen, A., Nordling, S., Hollmen, S., Eskelinen, M., Syrjanen, K. and Alhava, E. (1998) Clinical relevance of p53 index and expression of proliferating cell nuclear antigen and Ki-67 in gastric cancer. *J. Cancer Res. Clin. Oncol.* 124:497-502.

[53] Shibuya, M., Hoshino, T., Ito, S., Wacker, M.R., Prados, M.D., Davis, R.L. and Wilson, C.B. (1992) Meningiomas: Clinical implications of a high proliferative potential determined by bromodeoxyuridine labeling. *Neurosurgery* 30; 494-498.

[54] Simpson, D. (1957) The recurrence of intracranial meningiomas after surgical treatment. *J. Neurol. Neurosurg. Psychiatry* 20; 22-39.

[55] Tsutsumi, Y. and Fushiki, S. (2000) Comparison of cell kinetics between the boundary and the interboundary areas during hindbrain segmentation in the chick embryo. *Acta Histochem. Cytochem.* 33; 141-147.

[56] Wolfsberger, S., Doostkam, S., Boecher-Schwarz, H.G., Roessler, K., van Trotsenburg, M., Hainfellner, J.A. and Knosp, E. (2004) Progesterone-receptor index in meningiomas: correlation with clinico-pathological parameters and review of the literature. *Neurosurg. Rev.* 27:238-245.

[57] Yamasaki, F., Yoshioka, H., Hama, S., Sugiyama, K., Arita, K. and Kurisu, K. (2000) Recurrence of meningiomas. *Cancer* 89:1102-1110.

In: Focus on Brain Cancer Research
Editor: Andrew V. Yang, pp. 113-145
ISBN 1-59454-973-7

Chapter VII

The Significance of Immunohistochemistry in Brain Tumor Diagnostics and Immunotherapy

Bela Bodey*[*]*, Bela Bodey Jr. and Stuart E. Siegel

Department of Pathology, Keck School of Medicine, University of Southern California, Los Angeles, and Childrens Center for Cancer and Blood Diseases, Childrens Hospital Los Angeles, Los Angeles, CA, USA.

Abstract

Neoplastic transformation evolves over a period of time involving the progression of cellular immunophenotype (IP) from normal to hyperplastic to dysplastic, and finally, to fully malignant. Superimposed on these changes is the interaction of the initiated cell with its microenvironment, whereby the neoplastically transformed cells, through the regulation or dysregulation of cytoskeletal, integrin, protease and adhesion molecules among others, develop a novel manner of relation with their surrounding microenvironment. Studies of the neuroendocrine-immune network reveal that the hormonal and cytokine milieu plays an important role impacting the growth and dedifferentiation capabilities of cancer cells. This is further affected by the tumor cells themselves inasmuch as they determine and regulate the constitution of their hormonal microenvironment, allowing the most aggressive and invasive of neoplastically transformed cell clones to promote their own growth and dissemination.

This chapter details the clinical significance of immunohistochemistry that has developed over the last quarter century. The advancement of monoclonal antibody (MoAB) technology has been of great significance in ensuring the place of immunohistochemistry

[*] Corresponding Author: Bela Bodey, M.D., D. Sc., 8000-1 Canby Avenue, Reseda, CA 91335, USA, Phone and Facsimile: (818) 886-1082, E-Mail: Bodey18@aol.com

in the increasingly accurate microscopic diagnosis of human neoplasms, becoming a method of choice in neuropathology. Selected groups of target molecules of great significance in general cancer biology and of particular importance in brain tumors are discussed. The discovery of neoplasm associated antigens (NAAs) has not only made the more accurate diagnosis of human cancer feasible, but has also shed light on the extensive IP heterogeneity of even the most closely linked human malignancies. The identification of disseminated neoplastically transformed cells by immunohistochemistry has allowed for a clearer picture of cancer invasion and metastasis, as well as the malignant evolution of the tumor cell-associated IP. The sensitivity and significance of immunohistochemistry lies not only in the detection of various tumor-associated markers, but also in the use of information gleaned from extensive evaluations of a particular tumor in establishing a functional molecular biological, biochemical and humoral profile of the particular tumor. The elucidation of the steps of the progression of cancer from pre-malignant to invasive and metastatic forms is of utmost importance in the differential diagnosis of neoplasms and in the establishment of appropriate therapeutic regimens. These regimens will certainly begin to take on a more individualized form, targeting combinations of molecular markers in the increasingly more specific and efficacious management of brain tumors.

Key Words: Immunohistochemistry; Monoclonal antibody (MoAB); Cellular immunophenotype (IP); Cancer associated marker (CAM); Neoplasm associated antigen (NAA); Cancer/testis-antigen (CTA); Melanoma antigens (MAGE, BAGE, GAGE, and LAGE-1/NY-ESO-1); CTA-directed, individualized antineoplastic immunotherapy.

Introduction

During the last three decades, immunohistochemistry has revolutionized both the research and diagnostic endeavors of pathologists, including neuropathologists (1, 2). It is a great feeling to know that through our extensive research observations on brain tumors, which have been well documented in numerous articles, we have been able to contribute to these exciting developments. Certainly, the rapid advancement of MoAB producing technology has been of great significance in assuring the place of immunohistochemistry in the modern accurate microscopic diagnosis of human neoplasms, as a method of choice in histopathology. A conventional histopathologic diagnosis still relies on the microscopic morphological changes in the observed tissue slides. In the case of mammalian neoplasms, a number of structural changes characterize the specimen. These usually include a serious loss of normal tissue architecture, increased basophilia, variability of cellular shapes and nuclei, disproportion between cell nucleus and cytoplasm and a various degree of nuclear enlargement. Unfortunately morphologic cell and tissue changes that take place during the neoplastic transformation are highly variable allowing somewhat subjective evaluations by different pathologists. Certainly, the tissue changes that characterize neoplastic cell transformation are generally reduced to a neoplasm grading system. The worldwide employed grading system ranges from grades 1 to 4, with the larger numbers being assigned to more aggressive neoplastic behavior. It is the variability of neoplastic transformation that has led to the rapid development of immunohistochemical diagnostic procedures. Monoclonal antibodies (MoABs) have been employed in characterization of the fine antigenic structure of biological macromolecules. The technique take advantage of the important fact that MoABs react with a single antigenic epitope, rather than having an immunoreactivity representing an additive binding to heterogeneous antigenic determinants as is the case with polyclonal antibodies and conventional antisera. Employing certain, chosen libraries of newly developed poly- and monoclonal antibodies greatly improved the precision of microscopic diagnosis in histopathology and also the concordance between pathologists. Certainly, the most important principle of the evaluation of an immunocytochemical result in mammalian neoplasms remains that positive immunoreactivity is significant only when it occurs in neoplastic cells previously recognized by standard (usually the routine hematoxylin and eosin stain) microscopic morphology. However, it should be kept in mind that the evaluation of immunoreactivity is proper only when there is a concomitant interpretation of appropriate control slides. The importance of immunohistochemistry in cancer biology is certain, and the aim of this chapter is to describe some of the important contributions of this technique.

Brain Tumor Associated Markers

The main goal of molecular oncology during the 1980s and 1990s has been the discovery of a marker which would be specific for neoplastically transformed cells, as such, or for a neoplasm of specific tissue or organ differentiation line; and we have the feeling that this goal has not been fulfilled yet (3, 4). Presently, the literature consider a neoplastic marker as an increasing level of a substance which is not unique for neoplastically transformed or tumor cells, and is indeed expressed in normal cells. The marker could be localized in the cytoplasm of neoplastically transformed cells or on their surface. The marker may also be produced by the tumor-surrounding tissue (paracrine secretion) under the influence of the tumor cells. Therefore, the immunocytochemical results of identifying a tumor marker should be interpreted with great caution and should be always confronted with the results of routine histopathology, as well as other observations. This is valid even if the immunohistochemical results greatly improve the proper diagnosis and differential diagnosis. Immunohistological procedures should also be based on strictly standardized antigen detection techniques (5, 6). Histopathology and immunohistochemistry continue to be increasingly popular methods for predicting outcome in patients with malignant tumors. Recently traditional histopathologic studies have stressed the importance of endothelial proliferation in the diagnosis and prognosis of a wide variety of mammalian neoplasms. Immunohistochemical proliferation markers, in particular MIB-1, may be useful in assessing unregulated cellular behavior, whereas their role in establishing neoplastic cells is less clear. Similarly, numerous studies on p53 and epidermal growth factor receptor (EGFR) immunohistochemistry in mammalian neoplasm have demonstrated serious predictive values.

Advanced immunohistochemistry employs hundreds of well-characterized, highly specific antibodies recognizing only the desired, target antigens. The highly sensitive methods of immunocytochemistry have expanded our understanding of the biology and immunobiology of brain tumors (as well as a wide array of other tumor types) and have led to the development and refinement of ever more reliable ways of diagnosis and differential diagnosis of CNS tumors, among many others. WHO Histopathological Typing of Tumors by the CNS has shown progress for both the current members and possible new special types of brain tumors that may occur, especially for the meningiomas and neuro-epithelial/neuroglial type (7). The routine technique using light microscope examination was the most useful one for daily diagnosis for many years, but immunohistochemistry techniques are needed for difficult cases, *e.g.*, GFAP, NE 14, NSE, S100, and MBP. Diagnostic problems could be caused by tissue- or cell-sampling errors, which are influenced by the tumor location itself. Thus, neurosurgeons encounter problems with biopsy intraoperatives or with the mishandling of tissues.

Grading of CNS tumors must be put according to the clinical interest for further management of the patient. CNS grading ranges from grade I (benign looking) to IV (malignant). Morphological grading is based on Kernohan and Adson (8) or Kernohan and Sayre (9).

Classification and grading of astrocytic tumors has been the subject of several controversies and no universally accepted classification system is yet available. Nevertheless, acceptance of a common system is important for assessing prognosis as well as easy comparative evaluation and interpretation of the results of multi-center therapeutic trials. Besides WHO guidelines (10), the other systems of classification are the Kernohan, Daumas-Duport (SAM-A) (11), and TESTAST-268 (12). Karak and co-workers set out to evaluate each system in order to establish which one is the most useful (13). They reported the results of a single center study on comparative survival evaluation along with assessment of inter-classification concordance in 102 cases of supratentorial astrocytic tumors in adults. Hematoxylin and eosin (HandE) stained slides of these 102 cases were reviewed independently by two pathologists and each case classified or graded according to the four different classification systems. The histological grading was then correlated with the survival curves as estimated by the Kaplan-Meier method. The most important observation was that similar survival curves were obtained for any one grade of tumor by all the four classification systems. Fifty three of the 102 cases (51.9%) showed absolute grading concordance using all 4 classifications with maximum concordant cases belonging to grades 2 and 4. Intra-classification grade-wise survival analysis revealed a statistically significant difference between grade 2 and grades 3 or 4, but no difference between grades 3 and 4 in any of the classification systems. It is apparent from the results of this study that if specified criteria related to any of the classification systems are rigorously adhered to, it will produce comparable results. The group thus recommended that one system be adhered to because it would allow for objectivity and reproducibility. Their final recommendation was for the Daumas-Duport (SAM-A) system since it appears to be the simplest, most objectivized for practical application and highly reproducible with relative ease.

Molecular aspects underlying the differences of the subtypes of astrocytic glioma can also be used to classify these tumors. Godard and co-workers demonstrated that human gliomas could be differentiated according to their gene expression (14). The researchers found that low-grade astrocytoma have the most specific and similar expression profiles while primary glioblastoma exhibit much larger variation between tumors. Secondary glioblastoma display features of both other groups. We identified several sets of genes with relatively highly correlated expression within groups that: (a). can be associated with specific biological functions; and (b). effectively differentiate tumor class. Such classification techniques allow for the development of targeted treatment strategies adapted to individual patients and allow for patient stratification (15). Moreover, using a genetic classification approach, classification success rates of up to 89% accuracy have been obtained (16).

Immunohistochemical markers are also proving to be a useful tool for characterizing medulloblastomas (MEDs). Medulloblastomas occurring in children represent a histological spectrum of varying anaplasia and nodularity. In order to determine whether immunohistochemical markers might be useful parameters in subclassifying these neuroectodermal tumors, Son and co-workers studied 17 childhood MEDs, including nine diffuse/non-anaplastic, four diffuse/anaplastic, three nodular/non-anaplastic and one nodular/anaplastic subtypes (17). The expression of neural cell adhesion molecule (NCAM), nerve growth factor receptor (NGFR), neurofilament (NF), synaptophysin (SYN), glial fibrillary acidic protein (GFAP), S100, Bcl-2, and Ki-67 was investigated by employing the immunohistochemistry against specific antibodies. The study showed that NGFR, NF, GFAP and S100 were not detected in anaplastic subtypes of MEDs (0/5), while non-anaplastic subtypes were mainly expressed within the nodules. All 17 tumors were reactive for NCAM, SYN and Bcl-2. In addition, Ki-67 labeling indices for anaplastic subtypes (39.0 +/- 7.42%) were significantly higher than that of non-anaplastic MEDs (11.4 +/- 8.04%; $p < 0.0001$). These results suggest, according to the authors, that immunohistochemical markers are a useful adjunct in characterizing subtypes of pediatric MEDs. In fact, scrutiny of the cytological variation found among MEDs has recently led to the concept of the anaplastic MED, which overlaps the large-cell variant and appears to share its poor prognosis. In contrast, the MEDs with extensive nodularity, a distinctive nodular/desmoplastic variant occurring in infants, has a better outcome than most MEDs in these young patients, proving that cytological and immunocytochemical data are indeed very relevant (18). Perry conducted a similar study as Son and co-workers and found that MED grading based on anaplasia demonstrated a statistically stronger association with patient outcome than clinical staging. Therefore, histologic grading of MEDs seems warranted as a routine diagnostic aid (19). Classification of the MEDs histopathologically and according to profiles of molecular abnormalities will help both to rationalize approaches to therapy, increasing the cure rate and reducing long-term side-effects, and to suggest novel, more individualized immunotherapeutical treatments (20).

Assessment of angiogenic potential by measuring the blood capillary density in histological sections assumes that a 4 mm thick section is representative of whole human solid neoplasm's vascularity. The number of blood capillaries was nonetheless counted at 1.0 mm^2 microscopic field (brain tumor tissue at 200x magnification), choosing microvessel hot spots on immunocytochemical slides stained by MoABs against endothelial cell markers (21).

Fourth-Modality, Molecular Marker-Directed Treatment

Cancer associated markers (CAMs) are the biochemical and immunological counterparts of the morphology of mammalian neoplasms. The expression of an immunocytochemically defined CAM is also related to the tissue of origin and is not a random event. At the same time the expression of a CAM can also be related to the particular developmental stage of tissues and organs (22, 23). Rapid advances in immunohistochemistry have resulted in the characterization of hundreds upon hundreds of highly specific poly- and monoclonal antibodies, recognizing only desired target antigens, which are useful in the IP assessment of normal and neoplastic cells. During the past two decades, the use of MoABs against oncofetal, neoplasm associated, cell lineage specific, endothelial, and cell proliferation related antigens in the diagnosis and biological assessment of prognosis in neoplastic disease gained increased importance. A sensitive direct correlation exists between the expression of certain molecules and the development of an invasive, highly malignant IP of neoplastic cells, allowing for the occurrence of angiogenesis and metastasis (24-30). Metastatic spread is a major factor in the prognosis of cancer patients. Early detection and eradication of circulating neoplastically transformed cells prior to the tissue development of distant metastases could help to improve the prognosis of tumor patients after therapeutic primary tumor resection. Disseminated neoplastic cells have been detected in different body compartments employing cytological and immunocytochemical methods and, more recently, employing different molecular biological techniques. The most frequently studied body compartments are the bone marrow, peritoneal cavity, blood and lymph nodes, but other body fluids such as urine, bile, pancreatic juice and sputum have also been analysed (31). At all of these sites, neoplastic cells have been detected (32, 33). In embracing a multidisciplinary approach to the management of breast cancer (BC) patients with sentinel node biopsy, the surgical pathologist task is to screen sentinel nodes for possible metastasis (34). The consequences of missing sentinel node micrometastasis can directly influence treatment strategies, and this screening therefore has to be performed with more attention than usual. There is a great diversity in the histopathological work-up of sentinel nodes, with many centres employing additional observation methods such as immunohistochemistry, reverse transcription polymerase chain reaction or flow cytometry in addition to the obligatory haematoxylin and eosin staining.

The fact still remains that in order to properly assess any immunohistochemical reactivity used for differential diagnostic purposes, the target cells have to be identified as neoplastically transformed cells by routine histopathological techniques. Selected groups of target molecules of great significance in cancer biology are discussed. The discovery of neoplasm associated antigens has not only made the more accurate diagnosis of human cancer feasible, but has also shed light on the extensive cellular IP heterogeneity of even the most closely linked human malignancies. The identification of disseminated neoplastically transformed cells by immunohistochemistry has allowed for a clearer picture of cancer invasion and metastasis, as well as the evolution of the tumor cell-associated IP towards increased malignancy. Immunoassaying (immunoreactivity) is also capable of detecting specific infectious agents, from ordinary bacteria to spirochetes, fungi, parasites and especially viruses, as well as identifying possible causative agents of CNS diseases.

During our immunocytochemical observations of brain tumor cellular IP, we employed the immunohistochemical method of "antigen liberation" or "antigen retrieval" (35-40). In the first step, antigen retrieval was sometimes achieved by single or combined enzymatic digestion (ficin, pepsin, and trypsin from Zymed Labs., South San Francisco, CA, USA) prior to the primary antigen-antibody reaction. Heat induced epitope retrieval (HIER) (41, 42), as modified by us, was also employed. Antigen retrieval required immersion of tissue sections, in a Target Retrieval Solution (DAKO Corp., Carpinteria, CA, USA) and heating in a water bath (95ºC to 99ºC). No single antigen retrieval solution works best with all antigenic epitopes. Our method with citrate-based (neutral pH) solution worked well with most antibodies applied in this study that required such pretreatment. Heat (microwave) targeted antigen retrieval resulted in an increase of antigen detection for a number of MoABs, and we also noticed a serious increase of immunoreactivity (*i.e.* staining intensity).

Implications of Brain Tumor Immunohistochemistry

Histopathology and immunohistochemistry continue to be popular methods for predicting outcome in patients with malignant gliomas. Over the past two decades, we have employed an extensive panel of over 90 antibodies in cellular IP characterization of medulloblastomas (MEDs)/primitive neuroectodermal tumors (PNETs) and astrocytomas (ASTRs), using a sensitive, four-step, alkaline phosphatase conjugated immunohistochemical antigen detection technique. The following is the most characteristic IP in MEDs/PNETs: Synaptophysin, Chromogranin A, HLA-A,B,C, HLA-DR, Vimentin, TE4, TE7, TE8, TE15, AE1, AE3, TE3, CLA, UJ 308, Leu 2/a, Leu 3a/3b, NF-H, MAP-1, MAP-2, MAP-5, GFAP, EGFR, p53, HOX-B3, -B4, -C6, c-erb-2 (HER-2), c-erb-3 (HER-3), c-erb-4 (HER-4), Caspase-3, FasR, Survivin, CD105 (Endoglin), COX-2, IGF-R, MMP-2, -3, -9, -10, -13, and in ASTRs: GFAP, Vimentin, Tenascin, HLA-A,B,C, HLA-DR, CLA, UJ 308, UJ 167.11, A2B5, Thy-1, Chromogranin A, NF-H, TE7, Leu-2/a, Leu 3a/3b, c-erb-2, c-erb-4, p53, Caspase-3, -6, -8, -9, FasR, CD105, COX-2, IGF-R, MMP-3, -10, MAGE-1. Overall, childhood MEDs/PNET and ASTR cells display a heterogeneous IP, differentiated as well as immature neurofilament proteins are present in most of these tumors, as well as neuronal differentiation is always present in all cases. Recently, traditional histopathologic studies have stressed the importance of endothelial proliferation in the diagnosis of GBM. Immunohistochemical proliferation markers, in particular MIB-1, may be useful in assessing oligodendroglioma behavior, whereas their role in malignant ASTRs is less clear. Similarly, new studies on p53 and epidermal growth factor receptor (EGFR) immunohistochemistry in gliomas have demonstrated only limited predictive values. Nonetheless, the importance of immunohistochemistry in tumor biology is certain, and the rest of this chapter is devoted in great part to the important contributions of this technique.

In the last decade, there is increasing recognition of polyphenotypic high-grade malignancies in non-CNS tumor literature. Some of these tumors have been regarded as variants of PNET or as extrarenal malignant rhabdoid tumors (MRTs). Jay *et al.* have described two posterior fossa neoplasms, both of which displayed a "polyphenotypic" expression of neural, epithelial, myogenic, and glial markers, including synaptophysin, neurofilament, vimentin, glial fibrillary acidic protein, S-100, neuron-specific enolase, desmin, S antigen, MIC2, cytokeratin, epithelial membrane antigen, and carcinoembryonic antigen (CEA) (43). One tumor showed complex intercellular junctions, cytoplasmic intermediate filaments, well-developed rough and smooth endoplasmic reticulum and Golgi apparatus, cilia, and neurosecretory granules. The other neoplasm showed pools of glycogen, desmosomes, and tonofilaments. The histological and ultrastructural appearances were inconsistent with glioma, PNET, meningioma, ependymoma, choroid plexus carcinoma, sarcoma, germ cell tumor, and other tumors in the WHO classification. Although the polyphenotype raises the issue that these may represent variants of MRT or the atypical teratoid-rhabdoid tumor, the morphologic findings in the two cases were very dissimilar. The two cases presented by the authors underscore the problems in nosology and classification of polyphenotypic tumors of the CNS. This is particularly significant, as therapeutic protocols for PNET, MRT, and non-CNS polyphenotypic tumors are quite different.

Mixed gliomas have been difficult to define and subsequently diagnose due to the paucity of literature specifically examining this group of tumors (44, 45). Thirty mixed gliomas in which the minor glial component comprised at least 20% of the total tumor were observed: 20 oligoastrocytomas (OA) and ten malignant oligoastrocytomas (MOA). Nineteen patients were male (mean age 36 years) and 19 patients presented with seizures. The tumor was located in the frontal lobe in 17 patients and the temporal lobe in nine patients. The duration of preoperative symptoms in 25 patients ranged from five days to 14 years (mean 2.6 years). A mean follow-up of four years was available in 29 patients. Fourteen patients, seven with OA and seven with MOA, had recurrent tumor. One patient with MOA and four patients with OA (three with tumor progression and one with extensive leptomeningeal spread) died as a result of their tumor one to five years after diagnosis. Eighteen patients received chemotherapy and/or radiation therapy. Twenty-five tumors were immunostained with antibody to p53 protein. p53 nuclear staining was seen in 5/16 OA and 3/9 MOA. Immunoreactivity was observed only in neoplastically transformed astrocytes. One of the four patients who died with OA was p53 positive. Three recurrent MOAs were p53 positive. It was concluded that mixed gliomas most frequently occur in the frontal lobe and the majority of patients present with seizures; that there is no obvious association of p53 detection in mixed gliomas with tumor grade or behavior; and that similar to pure fibrillary astrocytomas, a subset of OA and MOA may be associated with p53 alterations.

Ganglioglioma is a rare, mixed neuronal-glial neoplasm of the central nervous system that occurs in young patients and has a benign clinical course (46). 27 specimens were studied by routine histochemistry, 21 specimens by immunochemistry, and 14 specimens were examined at the ultrastructural level by Hirose and co-workers in an attempt to define the immunophenotypic and morphologic features of ganglioglioma. The age of the 27 patients, 14 males and 13 females, ranged from 3 to 52 years (mean 22 years). The most commonly affected site was the temporal lobe (13 patients). Three patients experienced a local recurrence. Microscopically, the tumors were comprised of well differentiated, somewhat abnormal neurons as well as glial cells, the latter including astrocytes of fibrillary (59%) and pilocytic (41%) type. Scant mitotic activity was observed in 2 tumors (7%). Glial cells of all tumors were immunoreactive for glial fibrillary acidic protein (GFAP), S-100 protein, and vimentin. Ki-67 labeling indices ranged from 0.6 to 10.5% (mean 2.7%) and p53 labeling indices between 1.1 to 42.4% (mean 15.6%). Ki-67 and p53 labeling indices in recurrent tumors were significantly higher than those of nonrecurrent ones (p=0.036 and p=0.026, respectively). No examples of anaplastic transformation were encountered.

Immunohistochemically, many neuronal cells were positive for synaptophysin (100%), Class 3 β-tubulin (100%), neurofilament protein (90%), and chromogranin A (86%), in addition to S-100 protein (71%) and, occasionally, vimentin (24%). Ultrastructural characteristics of neuronal cells included the presence of numerous, 100-230 nanometer dense core granules within both perikarya and cell processes, well developed rough endoplasmic reticulum, microtubules within cell processes, and synapses associated with clear vesicles. Astrocytic cells usually contained abundant intermediate filaments; their cell membranes, when abutting the stroma, were covered by basal lamina. It is certain that gangliogliomas are comprised of well-differentiated neuronal cells and glial cells that are very often of pilocytic type. No cells with features intermediate between neurons and glia were observed. Neuronal cells are characterized by prominent neurosecretory features distinct from those of normal neurons in the central nervous system. Furthermore, higher Ki-67 and p53 labeling indices may indicate more aggressive behavior.

A recent study by Haapasalo et al. evaluated the feasibility and utility of Ultrarapid immunostaining of Ki-67 in astrocytomas (47). It was found that the Ultrarapid technique, a method that could be carried out on frozen sections in about 10 minutes, provided reactivity comparable to that achieved with standard immunohistochemistry of paraffin embedded slides using the MIB-1 antibody. Thus, the Ultrarapid technique could certainly be utilized in the intraoperatve diagnosis of gliomas as well as other tumors.

Nerve growth factor (NGF) is important to the survival, development, and differentiation of neurons (48). Its action is mediated by a specific cell surface transmembrane glycoprotein, nerve growth factor receptor (NGFR). NGFR expression was examined by immunohistochemistry in human fetal and adult adrenal medullary tissue, peripheral nervous system (PNS) neuroectodermal tumors (neuroblastoma, ganglioneuroblastoma, ganglioneuroma), pediatric primitive neuroectodermal tumors (PNETs) of the CNS, and CNS gliomas. Sixty-nine tumors in total were probed in this manner. Nerve growth factor receptor immunoreactivity was confined to nerve fibers and clusters of primitive-appearing cells in the fetal adrenal, and to nerve fibers and ganglion cells of the adult adrenal medulla; adrenal chromaffin cells were negative. In PNS neuroectodermal tumors, there was NGFR expression in tumor cells of 6 of 11 neuroblastomas and 6 of 6 ganglioneuroblastomas or ganglioneuromas. Thirteen of thirty-five CNS PNETs showed NGFR positivity. In most CNS PNETs, NGFR was restricted to scattered single or small groups of cells, but two tumors with astroglial differentiation showed much more extensive immunoreactivity. Most ASTRs (11 of 14) and all ependymomas (3 of 3) were intensely NGFR positive.

In an earlier observation, MED-L cells with the 75kD low-affinity nerve growth factor receptor (p75NGFR) and MED-H cells with the proto-oncogene tropomyosin receptor kinase product (p140trk) were isolated selectively from a parent MED-3 cell line derived from cerebellar MED by panning, and the interaction of NGF with these cell lines was analyzed (49). NGF treatment induced neuronal differentiation, growth inhibition, and tyrosine phosphorylation of p140trk in MED-H cells, but not in MED-L cells. The cells of MEDs express the functional NGFR, p140trk, which regulates their differentiation and growth.

In another study, positron emission tomography (PET) with the amino acid tracer L-[1-C-11]-tyrosine was evaluated in 27 patients with primary and recurrent brain tumors (50). Patients underwent either static (n=14) or dynamic PET (n=13), with quantification of protein synthesis rate (PSR) and tumor-to-background ratio. Findings were compared with histopathological findings. Primary brain tumor was proved in 22 patients histologically, as well as metastatic cancer of unknown origin, primary non-Hodgkin lymphoma, meningioma, atypical infarction, and vasculitis in one patient each. At PET, 20 of 22 primary tumors, the metastasis, and non-Hodgkin lymphoma were correctly depicted. A false-positive finding was obtained with the infarction, and the meningioma and vasculitis were not depicted. The calculated sensitivity was 92%; specificity, 67%; and accuracy, 89%. There were no statistically significant relationships between histologic findings, PSR, and tumor-to-background ratio. The results strongly suggested that L-[1-C-11]-tyrosine is a valid tracer for early diagnosis of brain tumors and allowed quantification of PSR. PSR was further measured in human brain tumors using L-[1-(11)C]-tyrosine PET, and the PSR was compared to histopathological parameters of intratumoral cell proliferation and protein synthesis (51). The authors observed 20 patients who had a positive brain tumor biopsy and who also underwent PET analysis. Formalin fixed, paraffin tissue sections were stained employing the MoAB MIB-1, targeted against the core Ki-67 antigen, and nucleolar organizer regions (NORs) were measured as argyrophilic NORs (AgNORs). The PSR was determined using a kinetic model. PSR (in nmol/ml/min) ranged from 0.44 to 1.99 (mean 0.97), Ki-67 labeling indices ranged from 0.9% to 33.5% (mean 9.5%) and AgNOR area (in mm^2/cm^2) ranged from 0.13 to 0.85. No relationship was found between PSR and Ki-67 labeling neither index nor AgNOR area. These results suggest that the PSR and the intratumoral proliferation, as measured by Ki-67, are two independent processes.

Deregulation of telomerase, a ribonucleoprotein polymerase that compensates progressive loss of telomeric $(TTAGGG)_n$ repeats during DNA replication, has been suggested to facilitate tumorigenesis and cellular immortality by providing unlimited proliferation capacity for cancer cells (52). The relationship between tumor proliferation activity and *in situ* expression of the telomerase RNA component was investigated in 46 human grade I to IV ASTRs. Heterogeneously distributed telomerase RNA expression was detected from all of the tumor samples as well as from normal human brain tissue. However, expression of telomerase RNA was significantly increased in highly malignant tumors (p=0.024) and in tumors that showed increased proliferation activity determined by MIB-1 immunohistochemistry (p=0.014). Interestingly, increased telomerase RNA levels were observed in a subgroup of grade II ASTRs that showed significant increase in proliferation activity (p=0.047), indicating that the telomerase RNA component is already up-regulated in the early stages of ASTR pathogenesis. Telomeric repeat amplification assays revealed telomerase activity in 4/6 GBMs and in 1 rapidly proliferating grade II ASTR. These results suggest that increased tumor proliferation activity triggers telomerase activation *via* mechanisms that involve increased production of the RNA component of telomerase.

Abnormal p53 detected by immunocytochemistry has been identified to be a predictor of poor disease outcome in a variety of human malignant neoplasms, including brain tumors (53-55). The role of p53 alteration in the pathogenesis of intracranial neuroectodermal tumors was observed by Ng and co-workers (56). Formalin fixed, paraffin sections of 196 brain tumors were employed in the study. The results demonstrated up to 40% immunoreactivity (presence of p53 alteration) in high grade ASTRs (AA and GBM). p53 alterations were also detected in 11% of well differentiated ASTRs. The extent of tumor cell immunolabeling also increased from the low to high grade ASTRs. Only rare cases of oligodendrogliomas and MEDs showed positive immunoreactivity, whereas ependymomas and choroid plexus tumors were uniformly negative. It seems that p53 alterations play a role in the immunophenotype progression of ASTR cells from low to high grade, as reported by us in a previous study (57). Small, anaplastic ASTR cells were the predominant cell type expressing aberrant p53 protein.

Glioblastoma multiforme (GBM), the most malignant neoplasm of the human CNS, develops rapidly *de novo* (primary glioblastoma) or through malignant cellular IP progression from low-grade or anaplastic ASTR (so-called secondary glioblastoma) (58). It was recently reported that mutations of the p53 gene are present in more than two-thirds of secondary glioblastomas, but rarely occur in primary GBMs, suggesting the presence of divergent genetic pathways (59). Primary and secondary GBMs were screened by immunohistochemistry for murine double minute 2 (MDM2) overexpression and by differential PCR for gene amplification. Tumor cells immunoreactive to MDM2 were found in 15/29 primary GBMs, but in only 3/27 secondary glioblastomas (p=0.0015). MDM2 amplification occurred in 2 primary GBMs, but in none of the secondary GBMs. Only 1/15 primary GBMs overexpressing MDM2 contained a p53 mutation. These results suggest that MDM2 overexpression with or without gene amplification constitutes a molecular mechanism of escape from p53-regulated growth control, operative in the evolution of primary GBMs that typically lack p53 mutations.

In another article, p53 and MDM2 oncoprotein expression was evaluated in paraffin-embedded tissues from 61 patients with CNS gliomas (53 ASTRs and 8 oligodendrogliomas) and related to proliferation-associated markers [*i.e.* proliferating cell nuclear antigen (PCNA), Ki-67, and nuclear organizer regions (NORs)], as well as epidermal growth factor receptor (EGFR) (60). The authors employed a library of MoABs including PC-10, MIB-1, DO-1, 1B1O and EGFR 113 and the colloid silver nitrate (AgNOR) technique. MDM2 and p53 were co-expressed in 28% of the glioma cases. A p53-positive/MDM2-negative cellular IP was observed in 15% and a p53-negative/MDM2-positive IP in 20% of cases. There was a positive correlation of p53 and MDM2 expression with grade and proliferation indices. Univariate analysis in the group of diffuse astrocytomas showed that older age, high histological grade, high PCNA labeling index and high AgNOR score were associated with reduced overall survival (p<0.05). p53 labeling index, Ki-67 labeling index, AgNOR score, as well as tumor location and grade influenced disease-free survival (p<0.05), whereas the only parameters affecting post-relapse survival were histologic grade and Ki-67 labeling index (p<0.1). Multivariate analysis revealed that age, radiotherapy, PCNA labeling index and p53 labeling index were the independent predictors of overall survival. p53, Ki-67, MDM2, and EGFR labeling indices, as well as grade and type of therapy were independent predictors of disease-free survival, and grade was the only independent predictor of post-relapse survival. The authors concluded that p53 and MDM2 labeling indices, as well as EGFR and proliferation marker (PCNA and Ki-67) expression represent useful indicators of overall and disease-free survival in diffuse ASTR patients.

Formalin fixed, paraffin embedded sections of 84 oligodendrogliomas (63 primary tumors, 21 recurrences), 21 GBMs with oligodendroglial growth pattern (15 primaries, 6 recurrences) and 17 mixed gliomas was observed for the presence of mutations in exons 5-9 by means of single stranded conformation polymorphism (SCCP), temperature gradient gel electrophoresis (TGGE) and direct DNA sequencing. In parallel, p53 protein accumulation was determined by means of immunocytochemistry (61). The percentage of mutations was found to be higher than previously reported (6/44 grade II oligodendrogliomas, 4/19 grade III oligodendrogliomas, 4/15 glioblastomas). In four cases, the mutations lead to distinct changes in the primary or secondary structure of the protein (cysteine ==> tyrosine, proline ==> leucine) and were associated with marked accumulation of p53 protein. A significant correlation between p53 protein accumulation and TP53 gene aberrations was found ($p<0.001$), although p53 protein accumulation was detected more often than TP53 gene anomalies, indicating that factors other than TP53 gene mutation may also lead to p53 oncoprotein accumulation in brain tumor cells. A significant correlation was found for p53 protein accumulation and tumor grade, but not TP53 gene mutations. In conclusion, evaluation of p53 protein accumulation reflected the clinical course of oligodendrogliomas better than the mere presence of TP53 gene mutations.

The *c-myc* protein, which has been reported as a transcription factor having an unclear but apparent dual role in promoting cell proliferation and PCD, may be related to the relative absence of necessary growth factors for producing growth arrest (62). The gene encoding p53 has been described as the most commonly disrupted gene in human neoplasms, suggesting a tumor-suppressor function for wild-type p53 (63-68). High levels of p53 are associated with arrest of the cell cycle in G_1, which allows for necessary repairs to be carried out following DNA damage and hypoxia (69). If the damage cannot be repaired, cell death by apoptosis is triggered. Mutations of the p53 gene lead to a loss of this critical DNA integrity and cell cycle monitoring function, which allows cells with damaged DNA to proliferate, obviously key in the production of neoplastically transformed cells. The bcl-2 family of proteins can inhibit (bcl-XL and Mcl-1) or induce (bax, bcl-XS, bcl-XL and bad) PCD in several cell systems (70-72). Bcl-2, a 25-26 kD protein, has been described in mitochondria, the nuclear envelope, and in the endoplastic reticulum. Recent data suggests that the activity of bcl-2 is regulated by a 21 kD protein bax, with extensive amino acid homology to bcl-2 (73). Bax is a homodimer capable of forming heterodimers with bcl-2. Bad is another protein that can interact with bcl-2. It has homology to bcl-2 within the homology domains BH1 and BH2. In mammalian cells, the bad protein is able to selectively heterodimerize with bcl-2 and bcl-XL, but not with other bcl-2 family related proteins. When bad is in a heterodimer with bcl-XL, it displaces bax from bcl-XL and promotes apoptosis.

Recently published evidence has emphasized the importance of PCD or apoptosis in the maintenance of tissue homeostasis and pathogenesis in the growth and progression of human neoplasms. This study, analyzed in breast cancer (BC), the significance of apoptosis in relation to the expression of p53 and bcl-2 proteins, tissue proliferation (defined by Ki-67 expression), hormone receptors, and tumor grade (74). Immunocytochemistry was performed for p53, bcl-2, estrogen receptor, progesterone receptor, and Ki-67 expression. Mutant p53 protein was detected using a mutant specific ELISA. Immunoreactivity of p53 significantly correlated with the presence of mutant p53 protein detected by ELISA ($r=0.654$, $p=0.00001$). An inverse correlation was observed between *bcl-2* expression and the extent of apoptosis ($r=-0.33369$, $p=0.01912$). The extent of apoptosis directly correlated with p53 protein accumulation ($r=0.485$, $p=0.00041$), Ki-67 immunoreactivity ($r=0.435$, $p=0.001$), histopathological grade ($r=0.492$, $p=0.0003$), BC size ($r=0.326$, $p=0.023$) and lymph node status ($r=0.287$, $p=0.047$). A direct correlation was also observed between p53 expression and Ki-67 immunoreactivity ($r=0.623$, $p=0.0002$). There was no statistically significant association between estrogen and progesterone receptor status and apoptosis. In addition, the TNM stage of the disease correlated with immunoreactivity of p53 ($r=0.572$, $p=0.00012$) and Ki-67 ($r=0.3744$, $p=0.00818$). Bcl-2, by inhibiting apoptosis, may cause a shift in tissue kinetics towards the preservation of genetically aberrant cells, thereby facilitating tumor progression. These results imply that rapidly proliferating tumors appear to have a high "cell turnover state" in which there may be an increased chance of apoptosis among the proliferating cells. The ability of apoptosis to also occur in the presence of mutant p53 protein suggests the existence of at least two p53-dependent apoptotic pathways, one requiring activation of specific target genes and the other independent of it.

Genetic observations have provided new insights into the regulation of developmental organization of PCD. During the development of the nematode *Caenorhabditis elegans*, two genes related to PCD were identified: ced3 and ced4 (two potential tumor suppressor genes), as well as, an inhibitor, a cell protector gene named ced9 (75-77). The ced9 gene is homologous to the bcl-2 proto-oncogene, discovered as a gene associated with a frequent translocation breakpoint in some B cell leukemias (78, 79). The ced3 gene encodes a cysteine protease that is homologous to the interleukin-1β-converting enzyme (ICE) (80). During the last few years, a number of novel genes involved in apoptosis, belonging to the ICE/ced-3 family and others, have been discovered: mouse Nedd 2 (81, 82), Ich-1, an ICE/ced-3 related gene that encodes both positive and negative regulators (83), TX/Ich-2/ICE_{rel}-II (84), the gene encoding CPP32, a novel human apoptotic protein with homology to the mammalian Il-1β-converting enzyme (85, Mch2 and Mch3 (86, ICE_{rel} II and ICE_{rel} III (87, ICE-LAP3 and ICE-LAP6 (88, 89), and MACH, a novel MORT1/FADD-interacting protease involved in CD95/*FasR*/APO-1, and TNF receptor-induced PCD (90). There is evidence that ICE family members are also auto-proteolytic, and are able to process one another's substrates, such as poly-ADP ribose polymerase (PARP), lamins, etc. (91-93).

Cadherins are Ca^{2+}-dependent cell adhesion molecules that play an important role in tissue formation and morphogenesis in multicellular organisms. In recent years, there have been reports of cadherin involvement in tumor invasion and metastasis (94). Twenty-two surgical specimens and some cultured cells were studied by immunohistochemical methods. No significant difference was observed in patients with AA, whereas decreased expression of N-cadherin was detected at the time of recurrence in those with GBM. In these groups, cerebrospinal fluid dissemination was found, and contralateral cerebral metastases and extracranial metastases were observed. It seems that decreased N-cadherin expression identified time of recurrence correlates with tumor invasion and dissemination of cerebrospinal fluid.

Desmosomes represent major intercellular adhesive junctions at basolateral membranes of epithelial cells and in other tissues (95). They mediate direct cell-cell contacts and provide anchorage sites for intermediate filaments important for the maintenance of tissue architecture. There is increasing evidence now that desmosomes in addition to a simple structural function have new roles in tissue morphogenesis and differentiation. Transmembrane glycoproteins of the cadherin superfamily of Ca^{2+}-dependent cell-cell adhesion molecules which mediate direct intercellular interactions in desmosomes appear to be of central importance in this respect. The complex network of proteins forming the desmosomal plaque associated with the cytoplasmic domain of the desmosomal cadherins, however, is also involved in junction assembly and regulation of adhesive strength.

Together with microtubules and actin microfilaments, approximately 11 nm wide, intermediate filaments (IFs) constitute the integrated, dynamic filament network present in the cytoplasm of metazoan cells. This network is critically involved in division, motility and other cellular processes (96). While the structures of microtubules and microfilaments are known in atomic detail, IF architecture is presently much less understood. The elementary 'building block' of IFs is a highly elongated, rod-like dimer based on an α-helical coiled-coil structure. Assembly of cytoplasmic IF proteins, such as vimentin, begin with a lateral association of dimers into tetramers and gradually into the so-called unit-length filaments (ULFs). Subsequently ULFs start to anneal longitudinally, ultimately yielding mature IFs after a compaction step. The assembly of nuclear lamins, however, starts with a head-to-tail association of dimers. Recently, X-ray crystallographic data were obtained for several fragments of the vimentin dimer. Based on the dimer structure, molecular models of the tetramer and the entire filament are now a possibility.

Tenascins (TNs) are a family of extracellular matrix glycoproteins. The first member of this family to be recognized, tenascin-C (TN-C), is known to be expressed in various tumors, including human ASTRs. Tenascin-X (TN-X) is the latest member of the TN family to be reported, and its expression in tumor tissues has not yet been examined (97). Expression of TN-X in glioma cell lines and human ASTRs was reported using immunoblot analysis employing anti-mouse TN-X antibodies. The expression pattern of TN-C and TN-X was also observed immunohistochemically in a series of 32 human ASTRs and tissue sections from five normal brains. Expression of TN-X was upregulated to a higher degree in low-grade ASTRs than in high-grade ASTRs. TN-X was mainly localized in the perivascular stroma around tumor vessels, and weakly expressed in the intercellular spaces among tumor cells. In contrast, TN-C was more strongly expressed in the intercellular spaces and in tumor vessels in high-grade ASTRs (AAs and GBMs) than in low-grade ASTRs. In the tissues expressing both TNs, the distribution of TN-X was often reciprocal to that of TN-C. These findings indicate that the expression of TN-C and TN-X in ASTRs is different, and that these glycoproteins could be involved in neovascularization in different manners.

Recent *in vitro* studies of the EGFR family have revealed complex signaling interactions involving the production of ligand-mediated heterodimers synergistic for the transformation of cells *in vitro* (98) and growth factors have been well established as necessary during the process of neoplastic transformation (99-102). In a series of 70 patients with childhood MED, immunocytochemistry and Western blotting analysis were conducted to characterize the expression patterns of all four EGFR family members (EGFR, HER-2, HER-3, and HER-4), as well as heregulin-α, a ligand for the HER-3 and HER-4 receptors. The majority of MED cases expressed two or more receptor proteins; coexpression of the HER2 and HER4 receptors occurred in 54%. Expression of heregulin-α was detected in 31% of the tumor cases observed by the authors. To investigate whether co-expression results in receptor heterodimerization, immunoprecipitation of protein extracts from primary tumors was conducted and various patterns of receptor interaction were observed, including that between HER-2 and HER-4. In multivariate 25-year survival analysis with clinicopathological disease features, no individual receptor or heregulin-α achieved significance. In contrast, when considered together in the multivariate model, co-expression of HER-2 and HER-4 demonstrated independent prognostic significance (p=0.006). These data suggest the hypothesis that HER2-HER4 receptor heterodimerization is of particular biological significance in MED, demonstrating the potential clinical significance of EGFR family heterodimerization in human neoplastic cells. The authors also analyzed expression of the AP-2 transcription factor implicated in the positive regulation of HER-2 and HER-3 gene transcription in malignant cells and found an association between AP-2 expression and not only HER-2 and HER-3, but also HER-4 levels in primary MEDs/PNETs.

The neurofibromatosis 2 (NF2) gene-encoded protein (merlin), may function as a molecular link between the cytoskeleton and the plasma membrane (103). Merlin is thought to play a crucial role as a tumor suppressor not only in hereditary NF2-related tumors, but also in sporadic tumors such as Schwannomas, meningiomas and gliomas. Using a merlin-expression vector system, specific antiserum against merlin was produced. Subsequently, the intracellular distribution of merlin in cultured glioma cells was observed, and merlin expression was further investigated in 116 human brain tumors. Immunofluorescence microscopy revealed that merlin was localized beneath the cell membrane and concentrated at cell-to-cell adhesion sites, where actin filaments are densely associated with plasma membrane. By immunohistochemistry, none of the Schwannomas from neither NF2 patients nor sporadic cases showed any immunoreactivity, while normal Schwann cells of cranial nerves were immunopositive. In meningiomas, merlin expression was frequently detected in the meningothelial subtype (8/10), but no expression could be detected in either the fibrous or the transitional variant. Most normal astrocytes were negative; however, reactive astrocytes often expressed merlin. Glioblastomas and AAs were found to be strongly positive, and focal positive staining was observed in fibrillary and pilocytic ASTRs. Thus, the loss of merlin appears to be integral to Schwannoma formation and the differential pathogenesis of meningioma subtypes. However, merlin alterations do not appear to play a critical role in neither the tumorigenesis nor the malignant transformation of neoplastic astrocytes.

Chang and co-workers have chemically characterized the gangliosides of the Daoy cell line in order to establish a model system for the study of ganglioside metabolism of human MEDs/PNETs (104). Cells comprising MEDs/PNETs contain a high concentration of gangliosides (143±13nmol LBSA/10^8 cells). The major species have been structurally confirmed to be GM2 (65.9%), GM3 (13.0%), and GD1a (10.3%). Isolation of individual gangliosides homogeneous in both carbohydrate and ceramide moieties by reversed-phase HPLC and analysis by negative-ion fast atom bombardment collisionally activated dissociation tandem mass spectrometry have allowed the authors to unequivocally characterize ceramide structures. In the case of GM2, 10 major ceramide subspecies were identified: d18:1-hC16:0, d18:1-C16:0, d18:0-C16:0, d18:1-C18:0, d18:1-C20:0, d18:1-C22:0, d18:2-C24:1, d18:1-C23:1, d18:1-C24:1, and d18:1-C24:0. Taken together with previous studies, these findings in human MED cells support the view that high expression and marked heterogeneity of ceramide structure are general characteristics of tumor gangliosides, molecules which are shed by tumor cells and are biologically active *in vivo*.

While the number of reports on macrophage infiltration of gliomas is increasing, the extent and mechanisms of macrophage recruitment remain unclear (105). To investigate whether monocyte chemoattractant protein-1 (MCP-1) plays a role in this process, *in situ* hybridization was performed for 22 GBMs, one AA and 4 grade II fibrillary ASTRs and reverse transcription-polymerase chain reaction was performed in 13 GBMs, one AA and three grade II ASTRs. High levels of MCP-1 mRNA were detectable in most GBMs, while a lower level was detected in grade II ASTRs. Many tumor-associated macrophages were observed by immunohistochemistry within most GBM cases, while the grade II ASTRs contained a lower number of infiltrating macrophages. The positive correlation between MCP-1 level and abundance of macrophagic infiltration suggests that MCP-1 has a role in the recruitment of macrophages to the site of the neoplasm. By combining *in situ* hybridization and immunohistochemistry, high levels of MCP-1 mRNA were shown both in tumor cells and within the tumor-associated macrophages. Reactive astrocytes and microglia along the boundary of the tumors also expressed MCP-1. In areas with T lymphocyte infiltration, larger numbers of MCP-1-positive cells with an enhanced level of expression were identified. The authors proposed that the mechanism of macrophage recruitment is, at least partly, affected by constitutive expression and T cell-mediated up-regulation of MCP-1 in tumor cells, as well as the tumor infiltrating macrophages. The production of MCP-1 by these macrophages establishes a positive amplification circuit for macrophage recruitment in gliomas.

In the last two decades, significant advances have been made in the identification of the soluble angiogenic factors, insoluble extracellular matrix (ECM) molecules and receptor signaling pathways that mediate control of angiogenesis (106). The question remains how the endothelial cells are capable of integrating these chemical signals with mechanical cues from their *in situ* tissue microenvironment so as to produce functional capillary networks that exhibit specialized form as well as function (107). These observations have revealed that ECM governs whether an endothelial cell will switch between growth, differentiation, motility, or apoptosis programs in response to a soluble stimulus based on its ability to mechanically resist cell tractional forces and thereby produce cell and cytoskeletal distortion. Transmembrane integrin receptors play a pivotal role in this mechanochemical transduction process because they both organize a cytoskeletal signaling complex within the focal adhesion and preferentially focus mechanical forces on this site. All three molecular filaments within the internal cytoskeleton (*i.e.* microfilaments, microtubules, and intermediate filaments) also contribute to the cell's structural and functional response to mechanical stress through their role as discrete support elements. A similar form of mechanical control also has been shown to be involved in the regulation of contractility in vascular smooth muscle cells and cardiac myocytes. The mechanism by which cells perform mechanochemical transduction and the implications of these findings for morphogenetic control are still not clear yet.

Experimental tumors of the CNS were observed with antibodies to quinolinate to assess the cellular distribution of this endogenous neurotoxin (108). In advanced F98 and RG-2 GBMs and E367 neuroblastomas in the striatum of rats, variable numbers of quinolinate immunoreactive cells were observed in and around the tumors, with the majority being present within tumors, rather than the brain parenchyma. The stained cells were morphologically variable, including round, complex, rod-shaped, and sparsely dendritic cells. Neuroblastoma and glioma cells were unstained, as were neurons, astrocytes, oligodendrocytes, ependymal cells, endothelial cells, and cells of the choroid plexus and leptomeninges. GFAP immunoreactivity was strongly elevated in astrocytes surrounding the tumors. Dual labeling immunohistochemistry with antibodies to quinolinate and GFAP demonstrated that astrocytes and the cells containing quinolinate immunoreactivity were morphologically disparate and preferentially distributed external and internal to the tumors, respectively, and no dual labeled cells were observed. Lectin histochemistry with Griffonia simplicifolia B4 isolectin and Lycopersicon esculentum lectin demonstrated numerous phagocytic macrophages and reactive microglia in and around the tumors, whose distribution was similar to that of quinolinate immunoreactive cells, although they were much more numerous. Dual labeling studies with antibodies to quinolinate and the lectins demonstrated partial co-distribution of these markers, with most double-labeled cells having the morphology of phagocytes. The present findings suggest the possibility that quinolinate may serve a functional role in a select population of inflammatory cell infiltrates during the host's immune response to primary brain neoplasms.

Cancer Testis Antigens as Targets

During the last decade, the aberrant expression of normal testicular proteins in neoplastically transformed cells became common knowledge. Cancer/testis-antigens (CTAs) represent a novel family of immunogenic proteins. The MAGE genes were initially analyzed from melanomas and turned out to have an almost exclusively neoplasm specific expression pattern. CTAs, were detected by serological screening of recombinant cDNA expression libraries. CTAs (*e.g.* members of the MAGE gene family) are a distinct class of differentiation antigens that have received much attention for being potential targets of human cancer vaccines for T lymphocyte based or receptor specific and directed immunotherapy because of their broad expression in various neoplasms (109, 110). The first member, MAGE-A1, of the MAGE gene family was discovered and characterized as genes encoding melanoma antigens (110). During the last decade, 23 human and 12 mouse MAGE genes have been isolated and characterized in various mammalian neoplasms (111). Numerous gene homologues to MAGE-A1 have been identified on the Xq28, Xp21,3 Xq26, and Xp11.23 and are classified as MAGE-A, -B, -C and -D (112-116). Previous observations have characterized the MAGE-A subfamily as: (a) they were not present in normal cells except for testis (primitive germ cells, spermatogonia) and placenta (117); and (b) some antigens encoded by the gene family are presented by the human leukocyte antigen (HLA) (118). These results suggest that immunoreaction against MAGE proteins could be expected to affect only neoplastically transformed cells (activation or derepression of normally silent CT genes) but not normal cells because testis and placenta lack HLA expression (119, 120). Melanoma antigens (MAGE) are regarded as inducing tumor-specific immune response and thought to be potential therapeutic agents for anti-neoplastic immunotherapy (121, 122). Hence, experimental vaccination with MAGE-A peptide provoked neoplasm regression in melanoma patients without significant side effects (109). The XAGE-1 gene consists of 4 exons and is located on chromosome Xp11.21-Xp11.22. The full length cDNA contains 611 bp and predicts a protein of 16,300 mol. weight, with a potential transmembrane domain at NH_2 terminus (123). XAGE-1 shares homology with GAGE/PAGE proteins in the COOH terminal. The XAGE-1b antigen, codes for a putative protein of 81 amino acids, harboring a functional bipartite nuclear localization signal and a C-terminal acidic transcription-activation-like domain. XAGE-1b has been shown to have a 50% homology with members of the GAGE family, at least on the nucleotide level (124).

Recently, a new CTA, NY-ESO-1 (one of the ten gene or gene families encoding CTAs), has been identified on the basis of spontaneous antibody responses to NAMs (125). NY-ESO-1 appears to be one of the most immunogenic antigens known to date, with spontaneous immune responses observed in 50% of patients with NY-ESO-1 expressing neoplams, inducing both a humoral immune response and specific $CD8^+$ cytotoxic T lymphocyte immunoreactivity (126-128). Immunity to NY-ESO-1 is clearly antigen dependent, disappearing with neoplasm removal or regression (129, 130).

A new member of CT genes, named OY-TES-1, was isolated and defined to be the human homologue of proacrosin binding protein sp32 precursor, which was initially found in the mouse, guinea pig, and pig (131). OY-TES-1, containing ten exons, maps to chromosome 12p12-p13, with Southern blot analysis suggesting that there are two OY-TES-1-related genes in the human genome. OY-TES-1 mRNA was expressed only in the testis when normal tissues were observed for its presence. However, OY-TES-1 mRNA was detected in various neoplastically transformed cells, including bladder, breast, lung, liver, and colon cancers. Ono *et al.* demonstrated through a serological survey of 362 cancer patients the presence of anti-OY-TES-1 antibody in twenty-five of these patients. In healthy individuals (n=20), OY-TES-1 sera reactivity was not identified, which indicates that these results show that the OY-TES-1 antigen is immunogenic in the course human neoplastic disease (132).

This expression pattern might contribute to the genetic instability of neoplastically transformed cells. Over the past few years, more than 200 research articles have appeared in the literature concerning CTAs (128). It has become obvious that CTAs can and will be used for the diagnosis and microstaging of various human neoplasms (129). Thus far, we have never seen authors writing about specific antigen families all arrive at the same conclusion, except in the case of CTAs, in which all authors have concluded that these antigens could and should be employed for more individualized, antigen targeted and specific anti-neoplastic immunotherapy.

Our immunocytochemical observations have detected the presence and cellular localization of the MAGE-1 CTA, employing anti-MAGE-1 MoAB, only in anaplastic, high grade ASTRs (100%) and in GBMs. The immunoreactivity was always heterogeneous, showing a cytoplasmic pattern and loosely grouped cells with similar staining characteristics being detected within the cellular and hormonal microenvironment of the ASTRs. MAGE-1 was not expressed in the lowest grade, pilocytic ASTR cases. The two cases of pure anaplastic ASTRs demonstrated expression of MAGE-1, located in the cytoplasm of neoplastically transformed cells. The staining intensity in this ASTR subtype was high (A and B) and the number of total cells positively stained ranged from (+) to (++). In the case of the *mixed* ASTR with primitive neuroectodermal tumor (PNET) elements, MAGE-1 was also present, but with a lower intensity (B) although a similar proportion of ASTR tumor cells exhibited immunoreactivity (++). No staining for PNET elements was identified. High intensity staining (A,B) in well over 50% of the total cell number (+++) was observed in the anaplastic oligo-astrocytoma and other anaplastic ASTRs. MAGE-1 immunoreactivity was of greatest intensity (A) in the four cases of GBM observed by us. A high proportion (over 50%) of the total cell number reacted positively (+++). Extensive immunocytochemical observations performed by our group have confirmed the expression of the MAGE family of peptides in numerous neoplastically transformed cell types including breast and lung carcinomas, and malignant melanomas. As expected, only some differentiating cells of the normal testis tissue, employed as positive tissue control in our immunohistochemical study reacted positively with the anti-MAGE-1 MoAB, while the other normal human tissues, including the postnatal thymus tissue demonstrated no detectable presence of MAGE-1 CT antigen (negative tissue controls).

Detection of Cancer/Testis Antigens in Various Malignant Neoplasms and Their Therapeutic Significance

It has become obvious that CTAs can be used for the diagnosis and microstaging of human neoplasms, as well as the population screening of smokers to show an increased risk for lung cancer in their own individual lifetimes and by extension, clearly showing the truly damaging effects of smoking. Thus far, we have never seen authors writing about specific antigen families all arrive at the same conclusion, except in the case of CTAs, in which all authors have concluded that these antigens could and should be used for antigen targeted and specific anti-neoplastic immunotherapy.

The expression of CTAs has also been examined in human brain tumors (133). Meningiomas were found to express only HOM-TES-14/SCP-1. SSX-4 was found to be the only CT gene expressed in oligodendrogliomas and it was also expressed in oligoastrocytomas and astrocytomas. Astrocytoma cells proved to be the most positive for HOM-TES-14/SCP-1 and SSX-4, with expression of HOM-TES-85, SSX-2 and MAGE-3 also defined in these tumors. MAGE-3 was detected only in grade IV astrocytomas, while the expression of the other CT genes showed no clear correlation with histological grade. Sixty percent of astrocytomas analyzed were found to express at least one CT gene, 21% expressed two CT genes, and 8% coexpressed three CT genes. These authors, like many others in relation to other neoplasms, concluded that a majority of oligoastrocytomas and astrocytomas might be amenable to CTA directed, specific immunotherapeutic interventions.

There has been observation of the expression of CTAs in cryo-preserved cutaneous T cell lymphoma (CTCL) tissues, including mycosis fungoides, pleomorphic cutaneous T-cell lymphoma, Sezary's syndrome (SS), and a non-malignant entity (small plaques parapsoriasis, SPP). The authors used a panel of eleven CT antigens (MAGE-1, MAGE-C1, MAGE-3, BAGE, GAGE, SSX-1, SSX-2, SSX4, SCP-1, NY-ESO-1 and TS85) (HOM-Tes-85), with mRNA expression for SCP-1 being identified in MF and pleomorphic CTCL patients but not in the small plaques parapsoriasis. SS patients demonstrated a more heterogeneous antigen expression pattern, including GAGE, MAGE-1, MAGE-3, MAGE-C1, NY-ESO-1 and TS85. Haffner *et al.* emphasized that CTAs could provide defined targets for antigen-based vaccination and CTA-directed immunotherapy in a high percentage of cases with CTCL. The authors also suggested that SCP-1 antigen expression might serve as an additional diagnostic indicator in early and clinically indistinct lesions suspicious for cutaneous T-cell lymphoma (134).

Another recent article by Mashino and co-workers analyzed the expression of six CT genes including NY-ESO-1, LAGE-1, SCP-1, SSX-1, SSX-2, and SSX-4 in gastrointestinal and breast carcinomas using reverse transcription-polymerase chain reaction (135). Relatively high expression of SCP-1 and SSX-4 was described in gastric carcinoma, LAGE-1 and NY-ESO-1 in esophageal carcinoma, and SCP-1 in breast carcinoma. Frequent synchronous expression with MAGE was identified, including LAGE-1 in esophageal carcinoma, SSX-4 in gastric carcinoma, and SCP-1 in breast carcinoma. Immunocytochemical analysis of the neoplasms expressing both MAGE-4 and NY-ESO-1 genes demonstrated differences in the distribution between MAGE-4 and NY-ESO-1 in serial sections. The authors suggested that NY-ESO-1, LAGE-1, SCP-1 and SSX-4, in addition to MAGE, genes may be promising candidates for NAM directed immunotherapy. The group of Mashino also added that polyvalent cancer vaccines may indeed be useful for cases of gastrointestinal and breast carcinomas with heterogeneous CTA gene expression profiles.

CTAs are also expressed in a high percentage in hepatocellular carcinomas. In 30 hepatocellular carcinomas, mRNA expression of SSX-1, SSX-2, SSX-4, SSX-5, SCP-1, and NY-ESO-1 has been described, with limited expressions of these genes being detected in few non-neoplastically transformed liver tissues (136).

Synovial sarcomas are high-grade, extremely malignant mesenchymal neoplasms with two, biphasic (BSS) and monophasic (MSS) variants that carry a pathognomonic cytogenetic alteration, t(X;18), involving the SYT gene on chromosome 18 and one of several SSX genes on chromosome X, usually SSX1 or SSX2, a translocation characteristically involving t(X; 18) to (p11.2; q11.2) between SYT and SXX (137). A recent study analyzed the expression of three CTAs, NY-ESO-1, MAGE-A1 and MAGE-C1 (CT7), through the use of immunocytochemistry, employing three MoABs, ES121 (anti-NY-ESO-1), MA454 (anti-MAGE-A1) and CT7-33 (anti-CT7), in synovial sarcomas (138). The results suggested that NY-ESO-1 is highly expressed in a homogeneous pattern in synovial sarcomas of both morphologic variants and both translocation types, making these neoplasms an attractive target for NY-ESO-1 antigen-based, and directed immunotherapy.

In the search for biomarkers for early lung cancer detection and possible receptor targeted immunotherapy, the frequencies of the expressional activation of MAGE-A1, MAGE-A3, and MAGE-B2 genes in non-small cell lung cancers (NSCLCs) were observed by Jang *et al.* (139). Expression of these genes was evaluated by reverse transcription-PCR (RT-PCR) in 20 primary NSCLC samples, with corresponding normal lung tissues, and in 20 bronchial brush specimens from former smokers without lung cancer. mRNA *in situ* hybridization was done to confirm the gene expression pattern at the cellular level. Among the twenty primary NSCLC samples analyzed, 14 expressed MAGE-A1 and 17 expressed both MAGE-A3 and MAGE-B2 while a substantial number of normal lung tissues adjacent to NSCLC also had detectable levels of MAGE expression, specifically 65% for MAGE-A1, 75% for MAGE-A3, and 80% for MAGE-B2. The activation of MAGE-A1, MAGE-A3, and MAGE-B2 genes was found to be common not only in NSCLC, but also in bronchial epithelium with severe carcinogenic insult. I agree with the authors that these results suggest that MAGE genes may be activated during the earliest stages of lung carcinogenesis, but more significantly, I feel that these genes should not only be considered as specific targets for lung cancer therapy, but that lung cancer prevention could be carried out *via* the population screening of smokers.

Since it has been both demonstrated and is now common knowledge that the MAGE genes are expressed in a wide variety of human neoplasms but only in the mitotic spermatogonia (germ cells) and in the primary spermatocytes in the normal testis, Aubry *et al.* chose to examine the expression of MAGE-A4 in a panel of testicular germ cell tumors (121). Classical seminomas uniformly and specifically expressed MAGE-A4 while anaplastic seminomas and NSGCTs were negative for this antigen. MAGE-A4 was also present in the fetal precursors of the stem germ cells from 17 weeks of gestation onward, which is in agreement with the fact that CIS can arise from prespermatogonia in the fetus. These results reveal that the MAGE-A4 antigen can be considered a specific marker for normal premeiotic germ cells and germ cell neoplasms and can in fact be employed as immunocytochemical markers to characterize classical seminomas.

The MAGE-3 gene is present in a variety of neoplasms, including lung cancer, but not in normal tissues except for the testis and placenta (140). The scientific aim of a recent observation by Eifuku and co-workers was to clarify whether HLA-A2 restricted MAGE-3 peptide (FLWGPRALV) was a lung cancer associated antigen recognizable by cytotoxic, $CD8^+$ T lymphocytes (CTL). MAGE-3-derived peptide-specific CTL were induced from the peripheral blood mononuclear cells (PBMC) of HLA-A0201-positive healthy donors and the regional lymph node lymphocytes (RLNL) of HLA-A2-positive patients with lung cancer by multiple stimulations with peptide-pulsed HLA-A0201-positive antigen-presenting cells. The lymphocytes stimulated with MAGE-3 peptide produced an antigen directed, specific lysis of Epstein-Barr virus-transformed B cells (EBV-B) pulsing with MAGE-3 peptide. Stronger and specific activity for MAGE-3-presenting targets was found after the second antigenic stimulation, and the activity increased with every repeated stimulation. The peptide-specific activity was inhibited by the addition of MoABs against MHC class I and HLA-A2. Such CTL also recognized established tumor cell lines expressing both HLA-A2 and MAGE-3 in an MHC class I-restricted manner, but did not recognize tumor cell lines that did not express HLA-A2 or MAGE-3. These results suggest that the MAGE-3 peptide could be used as a potential target for antigen directed, specific immunotherapy for HLA-A2 patients with lung cancer (140).

As neoplastically transformed cells spread beyond their primary site, they undergo changes in their gene expression that may be detectable and useful for microstaging of neoplastic disease (141). The CT antigens like MAGE 1-3, NY-ESO-1, SSX 1-5, and others are potential NAMs for microstaging melanoma. One CTA, CTp11, was shown to be expressed by metastasizing melanoma cell lines but not by nonmetastasizing variants. It was found that CTp11 tended to be expressed by primary melanomas. There was a statistically significant difference in the distribution of the expression of CTp11 and NY-ESO-1 in melanoma from different stages of progression. The authors concluded that NY-ESO-1 may be a prognostically significant CTA, detecting of more advanced neoplastic disease and CTp11 of less advanced disease.

Today it is well known that HLA-A*0201 melanoma patients can frequently develop a CTL response to the CT antigen NY-ESO-1. In a study by Romero *et al.*, the relative antigenicity and *in vitro* immunogenic effectivity of natural and modified NY-ESO-1 peptide sequences was analyzed (142). The results revealed that, although suboptimal for binding to the HLA-A*0201 molecule, peptide NY-ESO-1 157-165 is, among natural sequences, very efficiently recognized by specific CTL clones derived from three melanoma patients. In contrast, peptides NY-ESO-1 157-167 and NY-ESO-1 155-163, which bind very strongly to HLA-A*0201, are recognized less efficiently. Substitution of peptide NY-ESO-1 157-165 COOH-terminal C with a number of other amino acids resulted in a significantly increased binding to HLA-A*0201 molecules as well as in an increased CTL recognition, although variable at the clonal level. Among natural peptides, NY-ESO-1 157-165 and NY-ESO-1 157-167 exhibited good *in vitro* immunogenicity, whereas peptide NY-ESO-1 155-163 was poorly immunogenic. The fine specificity of interaction between peptide NY-ESO-1 C165A, HLA-A*0201, and T lymphocyte receptor was also analyzed at the molecular level employing a series of variant peptides containing single alanine substitutions. I agree with the authors that the results submitted in this article will have significant implications for the further development of NY-ESO-1 peptide based vaccines and for the monitoring of either natural or vaccine-induced NY-ESO-1 specific CTL responses in neoplasm patients.

The identification and characterization of L552S, an over-expressed, alternatively spliced isoform of XAGE-1 was reported in lung adenocarcinoma (143). Genomic sequence analysis has revealed that L552S and XAGE-1 are alternatively spliced isoforms, and expression of both L552S and XAGE-1 isoforms are present in lung adenocarcinoma. L552S was shown to be expressed at levels greater than 10-fold in lung adenocarcinomas compared with the highest expression level found in all normal tissues tested. L552S was present in both early and late stages of lung adenocarcinoma development, but it was not detected in large cell carcinoma, small cell carcinoma, or atypical lung neuroendocrine carcinoid. Immunocytochemical analysis employing affinity purified L552S polyclonal antibodies demonstrated specific nuclear staining in lung adenocarcinoma samples. Furthermore, antibody responses to recombinant L552S protein were observed lung pleural effusion fluids of lung cancer patients. These results strongly imply that the L552S protein is a strong immunogen and the authors suggested that it could be employed as a vaccine target for lung cancer (143).

In recent experiments of suppression subtractive hybridization, comparing mRNA expression profiles of common nevocellular nevi and melanoma metastases, was employed to identify new potential markers of melanoma progression (131). The metastatic melanoma tissues contained XAGE-1b. Expression of XAGE-1b in normal tissues was mainly restricted to testis, while placenta and brain were sporadically positive. In general, expression of XAGE-1b was much more prominent than expression of the longer XAGE-1 transcript, isolated from Ewing's sarcoma. In the different stages of melanocytic tumor progression, expression was exclusively seen in melanoma metastases, while all tested common and atypical nevi as well as primary melanomas were negative. Upregulation of receptor expression after treatment with demethylating agent 5-aza-2'-deoxycytidine was identified in only one of four human melanoma cell lines tested. After transfection of XAGE-1 gene into COS cells, the corresponding protein could direct the coupled fluorescent protein to the nucleus, showing a distinct speckled staining aspect. These experimental data imply the nuclear CT associated XAGE-1b to be a marker for late melanocytic tumor progression (131).

An extensive review of the expression of the SSX genes in a variety of human tumors has been provided by Tureci *et al.* (144). The authors assessed the expression of SSX-1, -2, -3, -4 and -5 using RT-PCR in a sample of 325 tumors of various histological origins. The expression of at least one of the SSX family members was found to be most frequent in cancers of the head and neck, followed by ovarian cancer, malignant melanoma, lymphoma, colorectal cancer and breast cancer while some leukemias, leiomyosarcomas, seminomas and thyroid cancers were found not to express any SSX gene. These findings further illustrate the amenability of CTAs for use in the targeting of various antigen specific immunotherapeutical approaches.

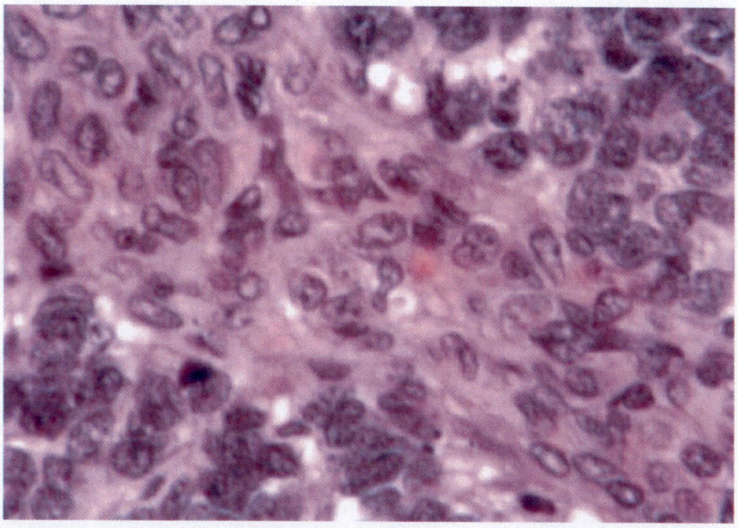

Figure 1. Childhood anaplastic ASTR. Expression of caspase-9 in the cytoplasm of neoplastically transformed cells. Routine, 10% buffered formalin fixation. Paraffin wax embedding. Alkaline phosphatase conjugated streptavidin-biotin antigen detection technique on a 4 μm thick section. Magnification: 500x.

Extensive immunocytochemical observations performed by our group have confirmed the expression of the MAGE family of peptides in numerous neoplastically transformed tissues including breast and lung carcinomas, malignant melanomas and childhood astrocytomas. Of particular significance is the absence of these markers on the surface of neoplastically non-transformed cells in normal tissues examined employing the same protocol, further substantiating the prevailing conclusions in regards to the specificity of the CTAs to genetically dedifferentiated populations of neoplastic cells and the distinct and very enticing possibility for their targeting in various immunotherapeutic approaches.

Conclusion

It has become clear that immunohistochemistry has revitalized morphological methods in cancer research and clinical oncology. As detailed in the foregoing discussion, the importance of this technique lies not only in its use in basic research focused on the mechanisms and regulatory steps in carcinogenesis, but also in its use in the more accurate diagnosis of neoplasia, including the functional differential diagnosis and staging of brain tumors. It has become clear that the evaluation of the expression of molecular markers of progression, invasion and metastasis should be employed routinely in the establishment of differential diagnosis and to aid in the determination of the most appropriate treatment regimen. The analysis of the IP expression profile of brain tumors of various stages has shed light on many possible NAAs that could be used as targets in fourth-modality immunotherapeutical approaches. It comes as no surprise, that the scientific conferences of the past decade demonstrated great interest in immunohistochemistry since this technique has allows researchers to delve into the molecular biological aspects of cancer, without sacrificing the tangible utility and beauty of morphology. The development of this technique to its present place in research, diagnostics and therapy, of course, could not have been possible without the discovery of monoclonal antibodies, one of the most important scientific discoveries of the twentieth century. The next 20 years will hopefully be increasingly dominated by the development of individualized "cocktails" of conjugated antibody molecules, targeting multiple antigens, as the main line of non-toxic and efficacious therapy of human cancer, especially in the treatment of residual and metastatic disease. With the advances made relevant to the genetic and molecular mechanisms of carcinogenesis it appears increasingly likely that etio-pathologic treatment will become a reality – that the treatment of cancer will be directed towards the etiology of the disease rather than just the symptoms and manifestations of the underlying pathologic process.

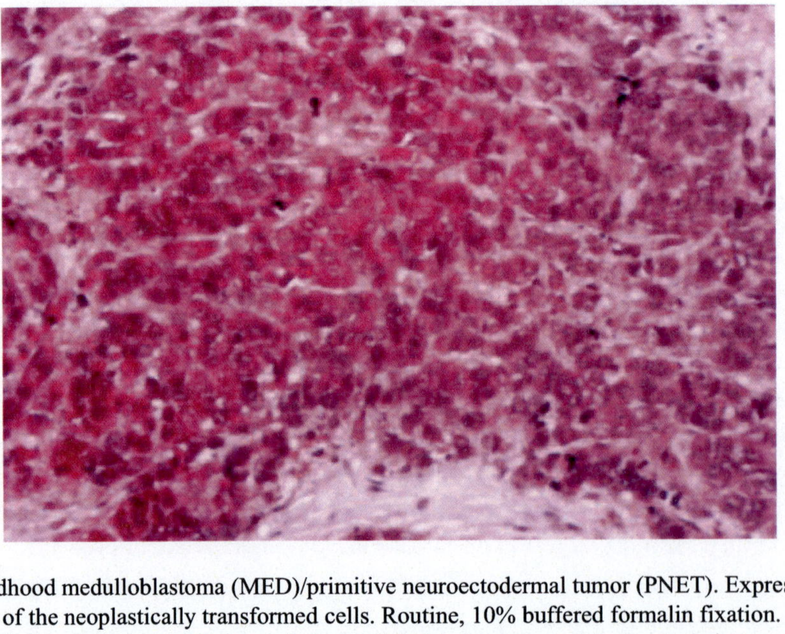

Figure 2. Childhood medulloblastoma (MED)/primitive neuroectodermal tumor (PNET). Expression of *FasR* on the surface of the neoplastically transformed cells. Routine, 10% buffered formalin fixation. Paraffin wax embedding. Alkaline phosphatase conjugated streptavidin-biotin antigen detection technique on a 4 μm thick section. Magnification: 200x.

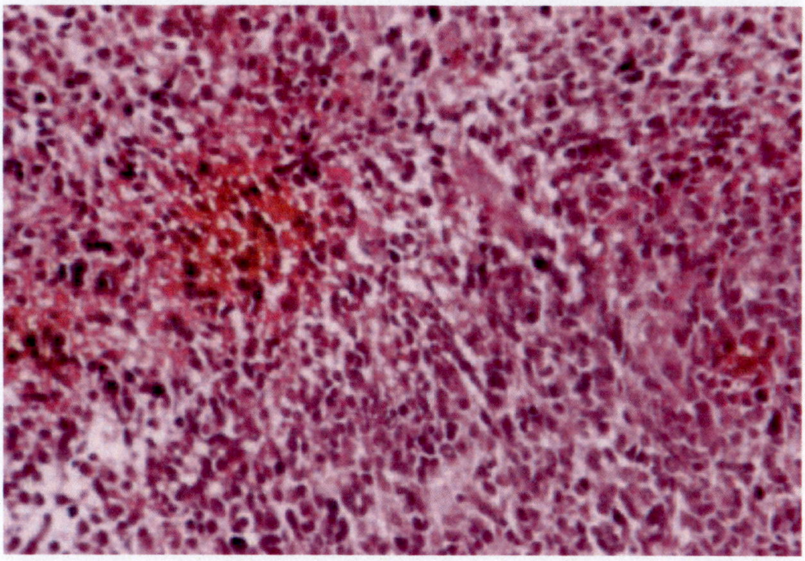

Figure 3. Childhood medulloblastoma (MED)/primitive neuroectodermal tumor (PNET). Expression of *FasR* on the surface of the neoplastically transformed cells. Routine, 10% buffered formalin fixation. Paraffin wax embedding. Alkaline phosphatase conjugated streptavidin-biotin antigen detection technique on a 4 μm thick section. Magnification: 200x.

References

[1] Kleinman GM, Zagzag D, Miller DC: Diagnostic use of immunohistochemistry in neuropathology. *Neurosurg Clin N Am* 5(1): 97-126, 1994.

[2] Miller CW, Simon K, Aslo A, Kok Y, Yokota J, Buys ChCm, Terada M, Koeffler HP: p53 mutations in human lung tumors. *Cancer Research* 52: 1695-1698, 1992.

[3] Szymas J: Diagnostic immunohistochemistry of tumors of the central nervous system. *Folia Neuropathol* 32: 209-214 1994.

[4] Husgafvel-Pursiainen K, Ridanpaa M, Anttila S, Vainio H: p53 and ras gene mutations in lung cancer: implications for smoking and occupational exposures. *J Occup Environ Med* 37: 68-76, 1995.

[5] Taylor CR: Quality assurance and standardization in immunohistochemistry. A proposal for the annual meeting of the Biological Stain Commission, June, 1991. *Biotech Histochem* 67: 110-117, 1992.

[6] Kawajiri K, Eguchi H, Nakachi K, Sekiya T, Yamamoto M: Association of CYP1A1 germ line polymorphisms with mutations of the p53 gene in lung cancer. *Cancer Res* 56: 72-76, 1996.

[7] Soetrisno E, Tjahjadi G: Pathological aspects of brain tumors. *Gan To Kagaku Ryoho* 27s(2): 274-278, 2000.

[8] Kernohan JW, Mabon RF, Svien HJ, et al: A simplified classification of gliomas. *Proc Staff Meet Mayo Clin* 24: 71-75, 1949.

[9] Kernohan JW, Sayre GP: Tumors of the central nervous system. In: *Atlas of Tumor Pathology*, Section 10, Vols 35 and 37. Washington DC. Armed Forces Institute of Pathology, 1952.

[10] Kleihues P, Burger PC, Scheithauer BW: *Histological typing of tumors of the central nervous system*. New York: Springer-Verlag, 1993.

[11] Daumas-Duport C, Scheithauer B, O'Fallon J, Kelly P: Grading of astrocytomas. A simple and reproducible method. *Cancer* 62: 2152-2165, 1988.

[12] Schmitt HP, Oberwittler C: Computer-aided classification of malignancy in astrocytomas: II. The value of categorically evaluated histologic and non-histologic features for a numerical classifier. *Analytical Cell Pathol* 4: 409-419, 1992.

[13] Karak AK, Singh R, Tandon PN, Sarkar C: A comparative survival evaluation and assessment of interclassification concordance in adult supratentorial astrocytic tumors. *Pathol Oncol Res* 6(1): 46-52, 2000.

[14] Godard S, Getz G, Delorenzi M, Farmer P, Kobayashi H, Desbaillets I, Nozaki M, Diserens AC, Hamou MF, Dietrich PY, Regli L, Janzer RC, Bucher P, Stupp R, de Tribolet N, Domany E, Hegi ME: Classification of human astrocytic gliomas on the basis of gene expression: a correlated group of genes with angiogenic activity emerges as a strong predictor of subtypes. *Cancer Res* 63(20): 6613-6625, 2003.

[15] Shai R, Shi T, Kremen TJ, Horvath S, Liau LM, Cloughesy TF, Mischel PS, Nelson SF: Gene expression profiling identifies molecular subtypes of gliomas. *Oncogene* 22(31): 4918-4923, 2003.

[16] Steiner G, Shaw A, Choo-Smith LP, Abuid MH, Schackert G, Sobottka S, Steller W, Salzer R, Mantsch HH: Distinguishing and grading human gliomas by IR spectroscopy. *Biopolymers* 72(6): 464-471, 2003.

[17] Son EI, Kim IM, Kim DW, Yim MB, Kang YN, Lee SS, Kwon KY, Suh SI, Kwon TK, Lee JJ, Kim DS, Kim SP: Immunohistochemical analysis for histopathological subtypes in pediatric medulloblastomas. *Pathol Int* 53(2): 67-73, 2003.

[18] Ellison D: Classifying the medulloblastoma: insights from morphology and molecular genetics. *Neuropathol Appl Neurobiol* 28(4): 257-82, 2002.

[19] Perry A: Medulloblastomas with favorable versus unfavorable histology: how many small blue cell tumor types are there in the brain? *Adv Anat Pathol* 9(6): 345-50, 2002.

[20] Ellison D: Classifying the medulloblastoma: insights from morphology and molecular genetics. *Neuropathol Appl Neurobiol* 28(4): 257-82, 2002.

[21] Rojiani AM, Dorovini-Zis K: Glomeruloid vascular structures in glioblastoma multiforme: an immunohistochemical and ultrastructural study. *J Neurosurg* 85: 1078-1084, 1996.

[22] Cairncross JG, Mattes MJ, Beresford HR, Albino AP, Houghton AN, Lloyd KO, Old LJ: Cell surface antigens of human astrocytoma defined by mouse monoclonal antibodies: identification of astrocytoma subsets. *Proc Natl Acad Sci* USA 79: 5641-5645, 1982.

[23] Rettig WJ, Nishimura H, Yenamandra AK, Seki T, Obata F, Beresford HR, Old LJ, Silver J: Differential expression of the human Thy-1 gene in rodent-human somatic cell hybrids. *J Immunol* 138: 4484-4489, 1987.

[24] Bodey B, Bodey B Jr, Gröger AM, Siegel SE, Kaiser HE: Clinical and prognostic significance of Ki-67 and proliferating cell nuclear antigen expression in childhood primitive neuroectodermal brain tumors. *Anticancer Res* 17: 189-196, 1997.

[25] Bodey B, Bodey B Jr, Siegel SE, Kaiser HE: Immunophenotypical analysis and immunobiology of childhood brain tumors. *Anticancer Res* 19: 2973-2992, 1999.

[26] Bodey B, Bodey B Jr, Siegel SE: Immunophenotypical (IP) differential diagnosis and immunobiology of childhood primary brain tumors. A decade of experience. *Int J Pediatric Hematol/Oncol* 6: 65-84, 1998.

[27] Bodey B, Taylor CR, Siegel SE, Kaiser HE: Immunocytochemical observation of multidrug resistance (MDR - p170) glycoprotein expression in human osteosarcoma cells. The clinical significance of MDR protein overexpression. *Anticancer Res* 15:2461-2468, 1995.

[28] Strojnik T, Lah TT, Zidanik B: Immunohistochemical staining of cathepsins B, L and stefin A in human hypophysis and pituitary adenomas. *Anticancer Res* 25: 587-594; 2005.

[29] Karim A, McCarthy K, Jawahar A, Smith D, Willis B, Nanda A: Differential cyclooxygenase-2 enzyme expression in radiosensitive versus radioresistant glioblastoma multiforme cell lines. *Anticancer Res* 25: 675-679; 2005.

[30] Purow BW, Haque RM, Noel MW, Su Q, Burdick MJ, Lee J, Sundaresan T, Pastorino S, Park JK, Mikolaenko I, Maric D, Eberhart CG, Fine HA: Expression of Notch-1 and its ligands, Delta-like-1 and Jagged-1, is critical for glioma cell survival and proliferation. *Cancer Res* 65: 2353-2363; 2005.

[31] Braun S, Pantel K: Diagnosis and clinical significance of disseminated tumor cells in bone marrow. *Dtsch Med Wochenschr* 125: 1237-1239, 2000.

[32] Vogel I, Kalthoff H: Disseminated tumour cells. Their detection and significance for prognosis of gastrointestinal and pancreatic carcinomas. Virchows Archiv 439: 109-117, 2001.

[33] Keene SA, Demeure MJ: The clinical significance of micrometastases and molecular metastases. *Surgery* 129: 1-5, 2001.

[34] Rampaul RS, Miremadi A, Pinder SE, Lee A, Ellis IO: Pathological validation and significance of micrometastasis in sentinel nodes in primary breast cancer. *Breast Cancer Research* 3: 113-116, 2001.

[35] Shi S-R, Key ME, Kalra KL: Antigen retrieval in formalin fixed, paraffin-embedded tissues: an enhancement method for immunohistochemical staining based on microwave oven heating of tissue sections. *J Histochem Cytochem* 39: 741-748, 1991.

[36] Shi S-R, Cote C, Kalra KL, Taylor CR, Tandon AK: A technique for retrieving antigens in formalin-fixed, routinely acid-decalcified, celloidin-embedded human temporal bone sections for immunohistochemistry. *J Histochem Cytochem* 40: 787-792, 1992.

[37] Key ME, Shi S-R, Kalra KL: Antigen retrieval in formalin fixed tissues using microwave energy. *US Patent # 5,244,787*; 14 September 1993.

[38] Beckstead JH: Improved antigen retrieval in formalin-fixed, paraffin-embedded tissues. *Appl Immunohistochem* 2: 274-281, 1994.

[39] Cuevas EC, Bateman AC, Wilkins BS, Johnson PA, Williams JH, Lee AH, Jones DB, Wright DH: Microwave antigen retrieval in immunocytochemistry: a study of 80 antibodies. *J Clin Pathol* 47: 448-452, 1994.

[40] Chen T, Zhang D, Shi S-R, Taylor CR: Antigen retrieval pretreatment: microwaving procedures and alternative heating methods. *BioLink* 4: 2, 1995.

[41] Shi SR, Cote RJ, and Taylor CR: Antigen retrieval techniques: current perspectives. J *Histochem Cytochem* 49: 931-937, 2001.

[42] Shi SR, Cote RJ, and Taylor CR: Antigen retrieval immunohistochemistry: past, present and future. J Histochem Cytochem 45: 327-343, 1997.

[43] Jay V, Edwards V, Halliday W, Rutka J, Lau R: "Polyphenotypic" tumors in the central nervous system: problems in nosology and classification. *Pediatr Pathol Lab Med* 17: 369-389, 1997.

[44] Beckmann MJ, Prayson RA: A clinicopathologic study of 30 cases of oligoastrocytoma including p53 immunohistochemistry. Pathology 29: 159-164, 1997.

[45] Krouwer HG, van Duinen SG, Kamphorst W, van der Valk P, Algra A: Oligoastrocytomas: a clinicopathological study of 52 cases. *J Neurooncol* 33: 223-238, 1997.

[46] Hirose T, Schneithauer BW, Lopes MB, Gerber HA, Altermatt HJ, VandenBerg SR: Ganglioglioma: an ultrastructural and immunohistochemical study. *Cancer* 79: 989-1003, 1997.

[47] Haapasalo J, Mennander A, Helen P, Haapasalo H, Isola J: Ultrarapid Ki-67 immunostaining in frozen section interpretation of gliomas. *J Clin Pathol* 58: 263-268; 2005.

[48] Baker DL, Molenaar WM, Trojanowski JQ, Evans AE, Ross AH, Rorke LB, Packer RJ, Lee VM, Pleasure D: Nerve growth factor receptor expression in peripheral and central neuroectodermal tumors, other pediatric brain tumors, and during development of the adrenal gland. *Am J Pathol* 139: 115-122, 1991.

[49] Kokunai T, Sawa H, Tamaki N: Functional analysis of trk proto-oncogene product in medulloblastoma cells. *Neurol Med Chir* 36: 796-804, 1996.

[50] Pruim J, Willemsen AT, Molenaar WM, van Waarde A, Paans AM, Heesters MA, Go KG,Visser GM, Franssen EJ, Vaalburg W: Brain tumors: L-[1-C-11]tyrosine PET for visualization and quantification of protein synthesis rate. Radiology 197: 221-226, 1995.

[51] de Wolde H, Pruim J, Mastik MF, Koudstaal J, Molenaar WM:Proliferative activity in human brain tumors: comparison of histopathology and L-[1-(11)C]tyrosine PET. *J Nucl Med* 38: 1369-1374, 1997.

[52] Sallinen P, Miettinen H, Sallinen SL, et al: Increased expression of telomerase RNA component is associated with increased cell proliferation in human astrocytomas. *Am J Pathol* 150: 1159-1164, 1997.

[53] Kyritsis AP, Bondy ML, Hess KR, et al: Prognostic significance of p53 immunoreactivity in patients with glioma. *Clin Cancer Res* 1: 1617-1622, 1995.

[54] Korshunov AG, Sycheva RV: An immunohistochemical study of the expression of the oncoprotein p53 in astrocytic gliomas of the cerebral hemispheres. *Arkh Patol* 58: 37-42, 1996.

[55] Bhattacharjee MB, Bruner JM: p53 protein in pediatric malignant astrocytomas: a study of 21 patients. *J Neurooncol* 32: 225-233, 1997.

[56] Ng HK, Lo SY, Huang DP, Poon WS: Paraffin section p53 protein immunohistochemistry in neuroectodermal tumors. *Pathology* 26: 1-5, 1994.

[57] Bodey B, Gröger AM, Bodey B Jr, Siegel SE, Kaiser HE: Immunocytochemical detection of p53 protein expression in various childhood astrocytoma subtypes: Significance in tumor progression. *Anticancer Res* 17: 1187-1194, 1997.

[58] Biernat W, Kleihues P, Yonekawa Y, Ohgaki H: Amplification and overexpression of MDM2 in primary (de novo) glioblastomas. *J Neuropathol Exp Neurol* 56: 180-185, 1997.

[59] Watanabe K, Tachibana O, Sata K, Yonekawa Y, Kleihues P, Ohgaki H: Overexpression of the EGF receptor and p53 mutations are mutually exclusive in the evolution of primary and secondary glioblastomas. *Brain Pathol* 6: 217-223, 1996.

[60] Korkolopoulou P, Christodoulou P, Kouzelis K, Hadjiyannakis M, Priftis A, Stamoulis G, Seretis A, Thomas-Tsagli E: MDM2 and p53 expression in gliomas: a multivariate

survival analysis including proliferation markers and epidermal growth factor receptor. *Br J Cancer* 75: 1269-1278, 1997.

[61] Hagel C, Laking G, Laas R, Scheil S, Jung R, Milde-Langosch K, Stavrou DK: Demonstration of p53 protein and TP53 gene mutations in oligodendrogliomas. *Eur J Cancer* 32A: 2242-2248, 1996.

[62] Packham G, Cleveland J: c-Myc and apoptosis. *Biochim Biophys Acta* 1242: 11-28, 1995.

[63] Clarke AR, Purdie CA, Harrison DJ, Morris RG, Bird CC, Hooper ML, Wyllie AH: Thymocyte apoptosis induced by p53-dependent and independent pathways. *Nature* 362: 849-852, 1993.

[64] Strasser A, Harris AW, Jacks T, Cory S: DNA damage can induce apoptosis in proliferating lymphoid cells via p53-independent mechanisms inhibitable by Bcl-2. *Cell* 79: 329-339, 1994.

[65] Glickman JN, Yang A, Shahsafaei A, McKeon F, Odze RD: Expression of p53 related protein p63 in the gastrointestinal tract and in esophageal metaplastic and neoplastic disorders. *Hum Pathol* 32: 1157-1165, 2001.

[66] Bodey B, Gröger AM, Bodey B JR, Siegel SE, Kaiser HE: Immunocytochemical detection of p53 protein expression in various childhood astrocytoma subtypes: Significance in tumor progression. *Anticancer Res* 17: 1187-1194, 1997.

[67] Bodey B, Bodey B JR, Gröger AM, Luck JV, Siegel SE, Taylor CR, Kaiser HE: Immunocytochemical detection of the p170 multidrug resistance (MDR) and the p53 tumor suppressor gene proteins in human breast cancer cells: Clinical and therapeutical significance. *Anticancer Res* 17: 1311-1318, 1997.

[68] Fuchs EJ, McKenna KA, Bedi A: p53-dependent DNA damage-induced apoptosis requires Fas-APO-1-independent activation of CPP321. *Cancer Res* 57: 2550-2554, 1997.

[69] Graeber TG, Osmanian C, Jacks T, Housman DE, Koch CJ, Lowe SW, Giaccia AJ: Hypoxia-mediated selection of cells with diminished apoptotic potential in solid tumors. *Nature* 379: 88-91, 1996.

[70] Naumowski L, Clearly ML: Bcl-2 inhibits apoptosis associated with terminal differentiation of HL-60 myeloid leukemia cells. *Blood* 83: 2261-2266, 1994.

[71] Reed JC: Regulation of apoptosis by bcl-2 family proteins and its role in cancer and chemoresistance. *Curr Opin Oncol* 7: 541-546, 1995.

[72] Haldar S, Basu A, Croce CM: Bcl-2 is the guardian of microtubule integrity. *Cancer Res* 57: 229-233, 1997.

[73] Oltvai Z, Milliman C, Korsmeyer SJ: Bcl-2 heterodimerizes in vivo with a conserved homolog Bax that accelerates programmed cell death. *Cell* 74: 609-619, 1993.

[74] Pillai MR, Kesari AL, Chellam VG, Madhavan J, Nair P, Nair MK: Spontaneous programmed cell death in infiltrating duct carcinoma: association with p53, BCL-2, hormone receptors and tumor proliferation. *Pathol Res Pract* 194: 549-557, 1998.

[75] Yuan J, Horvitz HR: The Caenorhabditis elegans genes ced-3 and ced-4 act cell autonomously to cause programmed cell death. *Dev Biol* 138: 33-41, 1990.

[76] Hengartner MO, Ellis RE, Horvitz HR: Caenorhabditis elegans gene ced-9 protects cells from programmed cell death. *Nature* 356: 494-499, 1992.

[77] Steller H: Mechanisms and genes of cellular suicide. *Science* 267: 1445-1448, 1995.

[78] Reed JC: Bcl-2 and the regulation of programmed cell death. *J Cell Biol* 124: 1-6, 1994.

[79] Pourzand C, Rossier G, Reelfs O, Borner C, Tyrrell RM: The overexpression of bcl-2

inhibits UVA-mediated immediate apoptosis in rat 6 fibroblasts: evidence for the involvement of bcl-2 as an antioxidant. *Cancer Res* 57: 1405-1411, 1997.

[80] Alnermi ES, Livingston DJ, Nicholson DW, Salvesen G, Thornberry NA, Wong WW, Yuan J: Human ICE/CED-3 protease nomenclature. *Cell* 87: 171, 1996.

[81] Kumar S, Kinoshita M, Noda M, Copeland NG, Jenkins NA: Induction of apoptosis by the mouse Nedd 2 gene, which encodes a protein similar to the product of the Caenorhabditis elegans cell death gene ced-3 and the mammalian IL-1β-converting enzyme. *Genes Dev* 8: 1613-1626, 1994.

[82] Sinkovics JG: Malignant lymphoma arising from natural killer cells: report of the first case in 1970 and newer developments in the FasL-->FasR system. *Acta Microbiol Immunol Hung* 44: 295-303, 1997.

[83] Wang L, Miura M, Bergeron B, Zhu H, Yuan J: Ich-1, an ICE/Ced-3 related gene, encodes both positive and negative regulators of programmed cell death. *Cell* 78: 739-750, 1994.

[84] Kamens J, Paskind M, Hugunin M, Talanian RV, Allen H, Banach D, Bump N, Hackett M, Johnston CG, Li P, Mankovich JA, Terranova M, Ghayur T: Identification and characterization of ICH-2, a novel member of the interleukin-1β-converting enzyme family of cysteine proteases. *J Biol Chem* 270: 15250-15256, 1995.

[85] Fernandes-Alnemri T, Litwack G, Alnemri ES: CPP32, a novel human apoptotic protein with homology to Caenorhabditis elegans cell death protein Ced-3 and mammalian interleukin-1β-converting enzyme. *J Biol Chem* 269: 30761-30764, 1995.

[86] Fernandes-Alnemri T, Litwack G, Alnemri ES: Mch2, a new member of the apoptotic Ced-3/ICE cysteine protease gene family. Cancer Res 55: 2737-2742, 1995.

[87] Munday NA, Vaillancourt JP, Ali A, Casano FJ, Miller DK, Molineaux SM, Yamin TT, Yu VL, Nicholson DW: Molecular cloning and pro-apoptotic activity of ICErelII and ICErelIII members of the ICE/Ced-3 family of cysteine proteases. *J Biol Chem* 270: 15870-15876, 1995.

[88] Duan H, Chinnaiyan AM, Hudson P, Wing JP, He WW, Dixit VM: ICE-LAP3, a novel mammalian homologue of of the Caenorhabditis elegans cell death protein Ced-3 is activated during Fas- and tumor necrosis factor-induced apoptosis. *J Biol Chem* 271: 1621-1625, 1996.

[89] Duan H, Orth K, Chinnaiyan AM, Poirier GG, Froelich CJ, He WW, Dixit VM: ICE-LAP6, a novel member of the ICE-Ced-3 gene family, is activated by the cytotoxic T cell protease granzyme *B. J Biol Chem* 271: 16720-16724, 1996.

[90] Boldin MP, Goncharov TM, Goltsev YV, Wallach D: Involvement of MACH, a novel MORT1/FADD-interacting protease, in Fas/APO-1 and TNF receptor-induced cell death. *Cell* 85: 803-815, 1996.

[91] Lazebnik YA, Kaufmann SH, Desnoyers S, Poirier GG, Earnshaw WC: Cleavage of poly(ADP-ribose) polymerase by a proteinase with properties like ICE. *Nature* 371: 346-347, 1994.

[92] Nicholson DW, Ali A, Thornberry NA, Vaillancourt JP, Ding CK, Gallant M, Gareau Y, Griffin PR, Labelle M, Lazebnik YA: Identification and inhibition of the ICE/CED-3 protease necessary for mammalian apoptosis. *Nature* 376: 37-43, 1995.

[93] Sorensen CM: Apoptosis or planning a death. *Biomedical Products* (September, 1996 issue), pp 38-39, 1996.

[94] Asano K, Kubo O, Tajika Y, Huang MC, Takakura K, Ebina K, Suzuki S: Expression and role of cadherins in astrocytic tumors. *Brain Tumor Pathol* 14: 27-33, 1997.

[95] Huber O: Structure and function of desmosomal proteins and their role in development and disease. *Cell Mol Life Sci* 60: 1872-1890, 2003.

[96] Strelkov SV, Herrmann H, Aebi U: Molecular architecture of intermediate filaments. Bioessays 25: 243-251, 2003.

[97] Hasegawa K, Yoshida T, Matsumoto K, Katsuta K, Waga S, Sakakura T: Differential expression of tenascin-C and tenascin-X in human astrocytomas. *Acta Neuropathol* (Berl) 93: 431-437, 1997.

[98] Gilbertson RJ, Perry RH, Kelly PJ, Pearson AD, Lunec J: Prognostic significance of HER2 and HER4 coexpression in childhood medulloblastoma. *Cancer Res* 57: 3272-3280, 1997.

[99] Aaronson SA: Growth factors and cancer. Science 254: 1146-1153; 1991.

[100] Engebraaten O, Bjerkvig R, Humphrey PA, Bigner SH, Bigner DD, Laerum OD: Effect of EGF, bFGF, NGF and PDGF(bb) on cell proliferative, migratory and invasive capacities of human brain-tumour biopsies in vitro. *Int J Cancer* 53: 209-214, 1993.

[101] Chicoine MR, Madsen CL, Silbergeld DL: Modification of human glioma locomotion in vitro by cytokines EGF, bFGF, PDGFbb, NGF, and TNFβ. *Neurosurg* 36: 1165-1171, 1995.

[102] U HS, Espiritu OD, Kelley PY, Klauber MR, Hatton JD: The role of the epidermal growth factor receptor in human gliomas: I. The control of cell growth. *J Neurosurg* 82: 841-846, 1995.

[103] Hitotsumatsu T, Iwaki T, Kitamoto T, Mizoguchi M, Suzuki SO, Hamada Y, Fukui M, Tateishi J: Expression of neurofibromatosis 2 protein in human brain tumors: an immunohistochemical study. *Acta Neuropathol* 93: 225-232, 1997.

[104] Chang F, Li R, Noon K, Gage D, Ladisch S: Human medulloblastoma gangliosides. *Glycobiology* 7: 523-530, 1997.

[105] Leung SY, Wong MP, Chung LP, Chan AS, Yuen ST: Monocyte chemoattractant protein-1 expression and macrophage infiltration in gliomas. *Acta Neuropathol* 93: 518-527, 1997.

[106] Guo P, Imanishi Y, Cackowski FC, Jarzynka MJ, Tao HQ, Nishikawa R, Hirose T, Hu B, Cheng SY: Up-regulation of angiopoietin-2, matrix metalloprotease-2, membrane type 1 metalloprotease, and laminin 5 gamma 2 correlates with the invasiveness of human glioma. *Am J Pathol* 166: 877-890, 2005.

[107] Ingber DE: Mechanical signaling and the cellular response to extracellular matrix in angiogenesis and cardiovascular physiology. *Circ Res* 91: 877-887, 2002.

[108] Moffett JR, Els T, Espey MG, Walter SA, Streit WJ, Namboodiri MA: Quinolinate immunoreactivity in experimental rat brain tumors is present in macrophages but not in astrocytes. *Exp Neurol* 144: 287-301, 1997.

[109] Boon T, Old LJ: Tumor antigens. *Curr Opin Immunol* 9: 681-683, 1997.

[110] Bruggen P van der, Traversari C, Chomez P et al.: A gene encoding an antigen recognized by cytolytic T lymphocytes on a human melanoma. *Science* 254: 1643-1647, 1991.

[111] Boel P, Wildmann C, Sensi ML et al.: BAGE: a new gene encoding an antigen recognized on human melanomas by cytolytic T lymphocytes. *Immunity* 2: 167-175, 1995.

[112] Ma Z, Khatlani TS, Li L et al.: Molecular cloning and expression analysis of feline melanoma antigen (MAGE) obtained from a lymphoma cell line. *Vet Immunol Immunopathol* 83(3-4): 241-252, 2001.

[113] Weiser TS, Ohnmacht GA, Guo ZS et al.: Induction of MAGE-3 expression in lung and

esophageal cancer cells. *Ann Thorac Surg* 71: 295-301; discussion 301-302, 2001.

[114] Chomez P, De Backer O, Bertrand M et al.: An overview of the MAGE gene family with the identification of all human members of the family. *Cancer Res* 61: 5544-5551, 2001.

[115] Ohman Forslund K, Nordqvist K: The melanoma antigen genes--any clues to their functions in normal tissues? *Exp Cell Res* 265: 185-194, 2001.

[116] De Plaën E, Arden K, Traversari C et al.: Structure, chromosomal localization, and expression of 12 genes of the MAGE family. *Immunogenetics* 40: 360-369, 1994.

[117] Rogner Uc, Wilke K, Steck E, Korn B, Poutska A: The melanoma antigen (MAGE) family is clustered in the chromosomal band Xq28. *Genomics* 29: 725-731, 1995.

[118] Lurquin C, De Smet C, Brasseur F et al.: Two members of the human MAGEB gene family loacted in Xp21.3 are expressed in tumors of various histological origins. *Genomics* 46: 397-408, 1997.

[119] Lucas S, De Smet C, Arden KC, Viars CS, Lethe B, Lurquin C, Boon T: Identification of a new MAGE gene with tumor-specific expression by representational difference analysis. *Cancer Res* 58: 743-752, 1998.

[120] Pold M, Zhou J, Chen GL et al.: Identification of a new, unorthodox member of the MAGE gene family. *Genomics* 59: 161-167, 1999.

[121] Aubry F, Satie AP, Rioux-Leclercq N et al.: MAGE-A4, a germ cell specific marker, is expressed differentially in testicular tumors. *Cancer* 92: 2778-2785, 2001.

[122] Gillespie AM, Coleman RE: The potential of melanoma antigen expression in cancer therapy. *Cancer Treat Rev* 25: 219-227, 1999.

[123] Chen Y-T, Old LJ: Cancer-testis antigens: targets for cancer immunotherapy. *Cancer J from Scientific American* 5: 16-17, 1999.

[124] Marchand M, Baren N Van, Weynants P et al.: Tumor regressions observed in patients with metastatic melanoma treated with an antigenic peptide encoded by gene MAGE-3 and presented by HLA-A1. *Int J Cancer* 80: 219-230, 1999.

[125] De Backer O, Arden KC, Boretti M et al.: Characterization of the GAGE genes that are expressed in various human cancers and in normal testis. *Cancer Res* 59: 3157-3165, 1999.

[126] Van Den Eynde B, Peeters O, De Backer O et al.: A new family of genes coding for an antigen recognized by autologous cytolytic T lymphocytes. *J Exp Med* 182: 689-698, 1995.

[127] Chen ME, Lin SH, Chung LW, Sikes RA: Isolation and characterization of PAGE-1 and GAGE-7. New genes expressed in the LNCaP prostate cancer progression model that share homology with melanoma-associated antigens. *J Biol Chem* 273: 17618-17625, 1998.

[128] Brinkmann U, Vasmatzis G, Lee B et al.: PAGE-1, an X chromosoma-linked GAGE-like gene that is expressed in normal and neoplastic prostata, testis and uterus. *Proc Natl Acad Sci* USA 95: 10757-10762, 1998.

[129] Brinkmann U, Vasmatzis G, Lee B, Pastan I: Novel genes in the PAGE and GAGE family of tumor antigens found by homology walking in the dbEST database. *Cancer Res* 59: 1445-1448, 1999.

[130] Liu XF, Helman LJ, Yeung C et al.: XAGE-1, a new gene that is frequently expressed in Ewing's sarcoma. *Cancer Res* 60: 4752-4755, 2000.

[131] Zendman AJ, Van Kraats AA, Den Hollander AI et al.: Characterization of XAGE-1b, a short major transcript of cancer/testis-associated gene XAGE-1, induced in melanoma metastasis. *Int J Cancer* 97: 195-204, 2002.

[132] Ono T, Kurashige T, Harada N: Identification of proacrosin binding protein sp32 precursor as a human cancer/testis antigen. *Proc Natl Acad Sci* USA 98: 3282-3287, 2001.

[133] Sahin U, Koslowski M, Tureci O et al.: Expression of cancer testis genes in human brain tumors. *Clin Cancer Res* 6: 3916-3922, 2000.

[134] Haffner AC, Tassis A, Zepter K et al.: Expression of cancer/testis antigens in cutaneous T cell lymphomas. *Int J Cancer* 97: 668-670, 2002.

[135] Mashino K, Sadanaga N, Tanaka F et al.: Expression of multiple cancer-testis antigen genes in gastrointestinal and breast carcinomas. *Br J Cancer* 85: 713-720, 2001.

[136] Chen CH, Chen GJ, Lee HS et al.: Expressions of cancer-testis antigens in human hepatocellular carcinomas. *Cancer Lett 164*: 189-195, 2001.

[137] Clark J, Rocques PJ, Crew AJ et al.: Identification of novel genes, SYT and SSX, involved in the t(x;18) (p11.2;q11.2) translocation found in human synovial sarcoma. *Nat Genet* 7: 502-508, 1994.

[138] Jungbluth AA, Antonescu CR, Busam KJ et al.: Monophasic and biphasic synovial sarcomas abundantly express cancer/testis antigen NY-ESO-1 but not MAGE-A1 or CT7. *Int J Cancer* 94: 252-256, 2001.

[139] Jang SJ, Soria JC, Wang L et al.: Activation of melanoma antigen tumor antigens occurs early in lung carcinogenesis. *Cancer Res* 61: 7959-7963, 2001.

[140] Eifuku R, Takenoyama M, Yoshino I et al.: Analysis of MAGE-3 derived synthetic peptide as a human lung cancer antigen recognized by cytotoxic T lymphocytes. *Int J Clin Oncol* 6: 34-39, 2001.

[141] Goydos JS, Patel M, Shih W: NY-ESO-1 and CTp11 expression may correlate with stage of progression in melanoma. *J Surg Res* 98: 76-80, 2001.

[142] Romero P, Dutoit V, Rubio-Godoy V et al.: CD8+ T-cell response to NY-ESO-1: relative antigenicity and in vitro immunogenicity of natural and analogue sequences. *Clin Cancer Res* 7: 766s-772s, 2001.

[143] Wang T, Fan L, Watanabe Y, Mcneill P et al.: L552S, an alternatively spliced isoform of XAGE-1, is over-expressed in lung adenocarcinoma. *Oncogene* 20: 7699-7709, 2001.

[144] Tureci O, Chen Yt, Sahin U et al.: Expression of SSX genes in human tumors. *Int J Cancer* 77: 19-23, 1998.

Index

A

B

C

D

H

I

J

K

L

M

N

O

P

Q

R

S

T

U

V

W